Handle With Care

Liane Jones

HANDLE WITH CARE

A Year in the Life of Twelve Nurses

MACMILLAN

First published 1995 by Macmillan

an imprint of Macmillan General Books
Cavaye Place London SW10 9PG
and Basingstoke

Associated companies throughout the world

ISBN 0 333 62925 6

Copyright © Liane Jones 1995

The right of Liane Jones to be identified as the
author of this work has been asserted by her in accordance
with the Copyright, Designs and Patents Act 1988.

All rights reserved. No reproduction, copy or transmission
of this publication may be made without written permission.
No paragraph of this publication may be reproduced, copied
or transmitted save with written permission or in accordance
with the provisions of the Copyright Act 1956 (as amended).
Any person who does any unauthorized act in relation to
this publication may be liable to criminal prosecution
and civil claims for damages.

1 3 5 7 9 8 6 4 2

A CIP catalogue record for this book is available from
the British Library

Phototypeset by Intype, London
Printed and bound in Great Britain
by Mackays, of Chatham plc, Kent.

For the nurses

Contents

Acknowledgements ix

Introduction xi

PROLOGUE
1

THE NURSES
8

THE YEAR AHEAD
28

WINTER
32

SPRING
124

SUMMER
199

AUTUMN
242

WINTER
285

EPILOGUE
335

Appendix 341

Index 343

Acknowledgments

My greatest debt of thanks is self-evidently to the nurses who appear in this book. I thank them for the honesty and imagination they brought to the project, and for their generosity in undertaking it in the first place. I'm also grateful for their good company – I enjoyed working with them very much.

I also owe thanks to 'St Alphege's' for allowing me to conduct my researches there. I should especially like to thank several people connected with St Alphege's who helped me with my research, answered queries and provided me with contacts. They must remain nameless here in order to protect others' identities; I know who they are, and I hope they do!

There are three people I can name who have given me valuable help with the book: Eve Jones and Jamie Buxton, who transcribed many of the tapes from my interviews, and Alan Jones, who carried out background research into diverse medical subjects and helped check the manuscript for accuracy. Their help allowed me to get to grips with the fascinating mass of material the nurses had provided.

I should also like to thank my agent Sara Fisher and my editor, George Morley, who was closely involved with the book at all stages of planning and writing.

Introduction

THERE ARE 630,000 qualified nurses in the UK today, and an estimated 400,000 of them work in the NHS. They work in hospitals, clinics, GPs' surgeries, nursing homes, schools and, increasingly, by visiting patients in their own homes.

Almost all of us have received nursing care at one time or another, even if it is only for a routine vaccination. Many of us will have had more prolonged contact with nurses – when we have been sick ourselves, or have been involved with family or friends who need nursing. We know what it is to rely on a nurse's judgement. Yet how many of us know what that judgement is based on and how far it extends?

What exactly are nursing skills and how do they differ from the things a doctor does? What happens when a nurse and a doctor disagree? What special skills are required before a nurse can work with mentally ill patients, with children or on an AIDS ward? These and other questions began to come thick and fast once I started researching this book.

Handle With Care is an attempt to look at nursing from the inside, and to give a picture of what life is like for nurses in the 1990s. It follows the working lives of twelve nurses throughout one year in the NHS. They are all connected to a large teaching hospital in London; some work in the teaching hospital itself, others in the smaller hospitals and specialist units associated with it. Seven of the nurses are students; five are qualified and working at various levels of seniority. In the course of the year their work will take us across the spectrum of nursing, from the technologically advanced AIDS speciality, to the overstretched and underfunded care of the elderly;

from therapeutic groups in mental health day units to emergency Caesarean births.

The nurses met me regularly to talk about their work, discuss their concerns and bring me up to date on events in the hospital; they also allowed me to accompany them on the wards and into staff meetings.

I owe them a huge debt of gratitude for their generosity, their patience and their willingness to talk candidly. I also extend heartfelt thanks for all the instruction in clinical and nursing matters they gave me along the way. With their help, I hope I have managed to avoid errors in the text – if any remain, they are my responsibility and I apologize for them.

Between them, the twelve nurses have provided me with a great mass of material. I haven't tried to give an inclusive account of their working year: it would be impossible, for they did far more than I have room to describe. Instead I have selected; I hope I have chosen rightly and managed to capture what they would consider most important.

St Alphege's is not the real name of the hospital. Every person and place mentioned in the book exists and all events described are real, but names have been changed throughout. I have changed details of the nurses' appearance and personal histories to protect their identities; I have similarly disguised the patients. In some chapters, I have altered the dates and times of events as a further precaution.

Prologue

IT WAS NOVEMBER when I began the interviews for this book and winter was settling in. Twelve nurses at St Alphege's hospital had agreed to let me follow them through the year ahead; I was waiting to meet the first of them in a steam-filled café on the corner of St Alphege's Square. Through the plate glass window and the rain I could see the hospital gates. A small crowd was gathering outside them. A furled banner was propped against the wall.

St Alphege's is one of the older and tattier of London's teaching hospitals. It stands in a busy part of the city, an island of soot-blackened brick around which cars, buses and vans roar or crawl, according to the time of day. Iron fire escapes sprout from the upper storeys. Tall windows allow light into cavernous wards. Visitors to the main courtyard may often be startled (and perhaps a little dismayed) to see a patient lying on a trolley, well muffled up against the cold, being pushed from one part of the hospital to another.

This institution was not built to meet the demands of modern medicine. However, meet them it has, and it now possesses an international reputation. Many of St Alphege's consultants are authorities in their fields; it has developed specialities in the treatments of AIDS, cancers and cardio-thoracic disorders. Within the old fabric of the buildings nestle some splendidly modernized facilities: seven new operating theatres built at a cost of £15 million; an AIDS ward with individual rooms; a resuscitation room, replete with state of the art equipment for saving lives.

All these things were under threat that November. Some time ago, the government had commissioned an investigation into health care in London. This had been carried out under the chairmanship of Sir Bernard Tomlinson; he had now just presented its findings in a report. The Tomlinson Report, as it at once became known, argued that London had too many hospitals duplicating one another's services and inadequate GP services. It proposed central planning for hospital provision in the capital, advocated that specialities like renal and cardiac units be concentrated in one or two hospitals per district, and earmarked several hospitals, large and small, for closure or for merger with their neighbours. St Alphege's was one of them.

The proposal to close Alf's took me – and most of Alf's staff – by surprise. We had all known that London's hospitals were under review but at the time St Alphege's didn't seem particularly vulnerable. The senior staff had been confident: this was a hospital of worldwide renown, after all. And it was not averse to progress: it was due to become a trust in the spring. Moreover, it was in the vanguard for nursing training. After years of government-backed consultation a new training course for student nurses had been devised: the government's ambition was that it would be taken up by all teaching hospitals in the UK by the end of the century. Eighteen months earlier St Alphege's had become one of the first London teaching hospitals to switch to the new training course, known as Project 2000. That was one of the chief reasons I was here.

Of the twelve nurses figuring in the book, seven were students. They were all eighteen months into their training, and represented the first generation of Project 2000 at Alf's. As such, they were pioneers – or guinea pigs, depending on the prevailing mood in the nursing college. For although little is known of Project 2000 outside the profession – and knowledge is patchy within it – it represents a decisive change in the way that nurses are trained.

The traditional method of training nurses in the UK is

to have them working on the wards from day one and learning as they go. This was the basis of the Registered General Nursing (RGN) course, operated by all teaching hospitals until recently: student nurses worked on the wards for three years with a programme of study running simultaneously. They had days off to attend lectures and do independent study; they wrote up projects over the course of the three years and also sat exams. At the end of the three years, if they had attained the required marks in the exams and projects, and if their ward reports came up to scratch, they became Registered General Nurses.* Meanwhile, they had already gained three years' experience on the wards, and had been counted in as members (albeit junior) of the hospital's workforce.

Project 2000 has shifted the emphasis away from learning on the job, giving a more academic bias to the training. It has been devised after years of consideration by commissions and professional bodies and it aims to 'professionalize' nursing. The idea is to give nurses a clear idea of their role in medicine (different from but not inferior to that of doctors). With increasing decentralization on the agenda for the NHS, Project 2000 is designed to prepare nurses to work autonomously, with wide-ranging responsibilities. Some would say that this is simply good nursing practice and already happens; on the whole, though, the clear statement that nursing is a profession as well as a vocation is welcomed by most.

Whether Project 2000, as it stands, provides the best training for this new, confident, professional nurse is a more contentious matter. Many people feel that there is too much time spent on theory and too long a delay before the students get out on to the wards for real, hands-on experience.

The first half of the course, lasting eighteen months, is called the Common Foundation Programme or CFP.

* Until the mid-1980s, the qualification was known as State Registered Nurse (SRN).

(Hospital life is full of initials.) It consists primarily of lectures and projects on basic biology and the pathology of human disease, together with a study of good practice in hospital and community nursing. There is a good deal of emphasis on the community, as it is the government's (and therefore the NHS's) stated aim to move resources from big hospitals into smaller units. These small units will provide medical treatment and nursing care on a part-time basis, with the patients staying at home. This is the crux of 'care in the community'.

During the CFP the students are sent out on to wards and into the community, on what are known as 'observation and participation' ('obspar') placements, to see how the theory is implemented. These placements are for observing and gaining some basic experience and take up only a small proportion of the students' time: for instance, on a five-week placement, a student might spend one day each week actually on the ward or with the community nurse, and the rest doing academic work; the students are not counted in as members of staff and are not expected to share the regular duties.

Herein lies one of the main differences between the RGN course and Project 2000. RGN students have always been 'student nurses', employed by the NHS to work as apprentices, whereas Project 2000 students are students and remain so until registration. They receive (low) bursaries rather than (marginally higher) wages. They get long student holidays for the first half of the course. For the duration of the CFP, at least, they are based in the college rather than on the wards and do not become part of everday hospital life.

Once the CFP is finished, the new course starts to resemble the RGN more closely, with an increased element of ward work. However, this is far from being the traditional across-the-board training, as Project 2000 now divides into four branches: Adult, Child, Mental Health and Mental

Handicap. Students must choose just one branch in which to specialize and they often have to choose in advance, before they start the CFP. Not surprisingly, this poses real difficulties for some students.

During the branch programme, the ratio of studying to placements is reversed. The next eighteen months consist mainly of work on the wards and in the community, with a certain amount of study running alongside. The exact make-up of the branch programme varies from one hospital to another. There are certain areas which must be covered under the Project 2000 remit; within that, each teaching hospital refines its branch programme to take advantage of its own circumstances.

One of the reasons that Alf's had become an early convert to Project 2000 was because its location and structure were well suited to the move. Like many large teaching hospitals, it was linked to a number of other units within the local health authority. It had a sister hospital, the Wavetree District General; it administered two smaller, specialist hospitals, the Markham for bowel disorders and St Wenceslas' Hospital for the elderly and mentally ill; and it had links with a range of community-based teams including health visitors, community nurses (the new name for district nurses) and community psychiatric nurses. This is a fairly typical spread of establishments for a teaching hospital – though most do not have the history and cachet of Alf's as well.

That November, the students had just emerged from the CFP into their branches. Since their enrolment, Project 2000 had become more widespread and was in place in almost half of the UK's teaching hospitals. At the time of writing, the changeover is near completion: although some RGN students are still working through their course, Project 2000 is in place in every institution that trains nurses and now constitutes the only way into nursing for new applicants. So the experiences of these first generation students at Alf's would also serve as an indicator of the way nursing is going.

Alongside the students, I was setting out to interview five qualified nurses. They too were all at Alf's or its sister hospitals, in different areas of nursing. They had varying lengths of experience and were employed at different grades – i.e. different levels of seniority. The grading system for nurses is complicated in detail, but the principle is that grades go from A (the lowest: usually a student nurse or 'support worker' with minimal training) to G (the highest: a nurse in charge of a large ward or a department, with management responsibilities), and each grade is paid within a certain range.

Students are A grades while they train. When they register they automatically become D grades. As such, they can be employed as staff nurses – a qualified nurse who is a regular member of hospital staff. As they gain experience, they can apply for jobs at a higher level, with more money and responsibilities. For example, senior staff nurse jobs are E grade; sister or charge nurse (the male equivalent title) posts are F. Thereafter, various kinds of sister/senior sister/ward manager titles proliferate, as nurses go up the hierarchy and progress to G grade. The appendix gives ENB (English Nursing Board) grades and rates of pay at the time of going to print.

That November, I was feeling my way into all this. I was acquainting myself with nursing terminology and getting to know the seven students and five qualified nurses who had volunteered to take part in the book. In the year ahead, I would be seeing them regularly and going on the wards with them, meeting their colleagues and their patients. By seeing their work through their eyes and listening to what they told me, I hoped to be able to give a reasonably vivid and accurate glimpse of nursing in the 1990s. But first, we were all trying to get the measure of what Tomlinson meant for Alf's.

On that wet, dark afternoon as I waited in the café to

meet one of the students, I realized that the crowd outside Alf's gates was a demonstration. The banner read 'Save Alf's – No to Closure'. Two nurses at the next table said there was to be a candlelit march to Trafalgar Square. Until now, I had been thinking of the nurses as twelve individuals and of next year as a chance to find out about their work at St Alphege's. Now it seemed that I would also be charting the hospital's fight to survive.

The Nurses

ANGELA TORRENCE was twenty-seven and American. She arrived at the café at a quarter past four, damp from the rain, and explained that she didn't have long because she was going on the march. She had a cup of coffee with suspicious-looking froth on it and gave me a quick history of herself.

She had not heard of Project 2000 when she applied to St Alphege's, she said. That had been three years earlier, when she had first come to London with her husband. I was surprised to hear that she was married. Somehow she looked single – an independent young American, dressed in very London 1990s style: thick leggings, boots, a woollen jacket. But it transpired that she lived in a flat south of the river with her husband Mark. He was also American, a theatre set designer and some years older than Angela; he had wanted to work in Europe, where opportunities for set designers are more plentiful than in the United States, and Angela had come with him.

Angela talked efficiently about herself; she was articulate and self-possessed. Her age contributed to this, of course – at twenty-seven, she was at the older end of the range for nursing students – as did the fact that she had experience of two cultures. She described herself as reasonably Anglophile: she liked many things about Britain, including the awareness of community that exists here; she disliked the administrative chaos that often accompanies it. Already, she said, she was coming to feel that the NHS exemplified this.

Angela intended to become a midwife. She was quite clear about this: she had made up her mind at fifteen, after a school visit to a maternity unit. Since then she had graduated from school, studied languages at university, lived in New York, married and moved to Britain, and throughout all these changes the idea of midwifery had kept its appeal. 'I like the idea of working with women, and with well women. Pregnant women aren't sick; pregnancy is a natural process and as a midwife you work with the women to help them keep healthy and have the best outcome.'

In this country, anyone wanting to be a midwife must first qualify as a nurse. Knowing St Alphege's by reputation and believing that an Alf's qualification would stand her in good stead both here and in America, Angela applied for the RGN course. Alf's wrote back, saying that they were due to implement Project 2000 soon and invited her to apply for that instead. Angela was more than willing: she didn't want to do a training that would soon become obsolete and she liked the fact that the Project 2000 course would equip her with a diploma in nursing rather than the old-fashioned certificate. She and her husband were likely to return to America in a few years' time and a diploma would be a solid qualification to take back. The only problem was that she would have to wait eighteen months, because Alf's was only just setting up the course. So she applied for the adult branch (an adult nursing qualification is compulsory for midwifery training) and waited.

Now, three years on, she was – 'Finally!' – on her first working placement. She spent two or three days each week on an elderly ward, interspersed with college days, and she was expected to work rather than just observe. At last she felt she was beginning to get some real nursing experience.

The CFP, in Angela's view, had taken a long time to teach the students very little. This was partly to do with the way the course was paced, but there had also been serious problems with its day-to-day administration. 'The teachers were just so unreliable. There were weeks at a time when the lectures were cancelled, moved, postponed – we would turn up and sit in an empty room, waiting for the teacher to show. Sometimes they wouldn't arrive at all; sometimes a message would come telling us the lecture had been put back to another day. It was such a waste of our time – I'd go home and feel like screaming with frustration.'

Days on placement had been keenly anticipated by all the students during the CFP, but there were difficulties there too. Staff on the wards had known little about Project 2000; they were unsure exactly what they were expected to do with the students and there was some resentment towards them. 'Some of the staff felt we were being babied. They'd say: "When I was a student I was thrown in at the deep end." ' Angela thought they had a point.

Like many of the other students, she had quietly registered with a nursing agency and topped up her bursary by doing a few days' agency work here and there on St Alphege's wards. The students were employed as 'A grades', the most junior level of nurse; even so, the experience had dismayed them. 'We realized how little we could actually do. And there we were, in our second year – it made us feel completely useless.'

It was clear that the sense of helplessness galled Angela. She mentioned it several times during that first conversation, in connection with college, the wards and her student status. In response, she had become active on the Student Representative Council and had been elected its chairperson last summer. The council did not have a particularly high profile; she and her colleagues on it were trying to change that and had raised several matters with the college already. Part of the problem, I gathered, was motivating other students to speak up.

Angela was cautiously optimistic about the year ahead. It was good to be on the wards, although she was finding the elderly ward gruelling: 'There's so much dementia. I find it difficult to cope with the destruction of the personality and the frustration of the patients as they try to communicate.' Her next placement would be maternity and she was looking forward to it, though, again, cautiously. A lot, she said, would depend on the staff and their attitude towards students. I had the distinct impression that as far as Angela was concerned the jury was out and would remain so for some time yet, not only on the course at Alf's, but on nursing as a whole.

OF THE SEVEN students I was to follow through 1993, five were on the adult branch; one was specializing in mental health (or psychiatric nursing, as it's often known), one in children's (paediatric) nursing. This reflected choices across the intake as a whole: at the end of the CFP sixty had gone into the adult branch, ten into the child branch and only eight into mental health. The adult branch was popular because it covered by far the widest range of medicine. Students interested in areas like cancer nursing, accident and emergency or midwifery needed to qualify in that branch; those without definite preferences selected it in order to keep their options open.

Emily Mallinson was one of the latter. A quiet young woman of twenty-four, she had left a job as a veterinary nurse because she found it too limiting, and her inclination was to get as broad a training as possible. Through her observation placements on the CFP she had discovered a leaning towards the elderly and she thought she might be interested in palliative care – nursing those for whom no cure was possible, such as cancer patients or people with AIDS.

Emily is very slight with a fine, sharp-boned face and a thoughtful manner which at first I misinterpreted as diffident. She was born and brought up in the south of England and had a boyfriend of several years' standing, Patrick, who lived in Hampshire.

I met her in her room in the nurses' hostel attached to St Wenceslas' Hospital, four miles to the east of St Alphege's, and off the tube map. The nurses' home is a modern red-brick block with a blank-faced look. It stands six storeys high, just behind the Victorian buildings that make up the bulk of the hospital. St Wenceslas had been due for redevelopment for years; successive plans had been drawn up and approved but somehow the money was never found. The elderly and mentally ill residents went on living in unsuitable wards which the staff made as comfortable and bright as they could – a daunting task.

Given its unpromising location, the nurses' home is not bad inside. It has a cheerful institutional air; the corridors are carpeted (hardwearing cord), the walls are painted pastel colours and many of the (admittedly tiny) rooms look out on to a pleasant garden.

There were 500 students and staff nurses living here. Emily's room was on the sixth floor with a garden view, but when I first visited it was night and the curtains were drawn against the cold. Emily was in jeans and a white shirt, buttoned up to the neck; she sat on the bed and talked seriously about nursing.

She had found the CFP interesting, particularly the emphasis on holistic care: dealing with patients as people. 'We've done a lot of psychology and sociology, just learning how to be with people and put their needs first, above the institution of the hospital. To some extent that's quite a new idea.

'When I decided to do nursing some people asked me why I didn't want to be a doctor instead. But that's totally crazy because a doctor does one thing and a nurse does something else. Doctors work on something called a medical model – they look at the disease and the condition and they treat them and try to cure them, whereas nurses work on a health model – you look on the person in terms of what health they can attain and what that health means to them, rather than just as someone in Bed 22 with a liver problem. On the CFP they taught us that we're supposed to look at people holistically. Not only have they got physical needs but social, spiritual and emotional needs and they live in the context of who they are, their family, their lifestyle. All that's going to affect how they respond to the illness they have.'

Emily found all this very encouraging. The holistic approach chimed with her personal, Christian, beliefs. Having started the course with a vague, old-fashioned notion that doctors gave nurses instructions, she was also pleased to find that she was expected to take responsibility for patients: – 'Though I hadn't expected all the regulations and pressures, and how that governs the way you nurse. We're always accountable for everything we do. There's a lot of form signing and monitoring involved.'

For all her quiet demeanour, Emily turned out to be a good, vivid talker. She was interested in the patients who had come her way so far and it was obvious that some of them, especially the older ones, had taken to her. She had stories of what people had said to her and in front of her. The memory of one patient in particular had stayed with her: a young man in his early twenties who was in a coma following a motorbike accident. 'I knew he wasn't likely to survive it and scans had shown that if he did, he'd be quite badly brain damaged. His mother was very, very distressed and not accepting at all the extent of damage he had or the likelihood that he wouldn't survive. And I found it very difficult to go into that room when I knew she was there and listen to her telling her son: "This is the day you're going to wake up. Come on, I know you're going to do it, I know you can hear me." Because he did have an awful lot of involuntary movement – twitching and hand-squeezing. Any new movement and she would say "Isn't that good?" I knew nothing about the likely course of his deterioration or what would be the signs of improvement, so I found it difficult to answer. I sometimes used to say "I don't know" or I would just smile. I used to talk to her instead about him – what kind of job he had, what he liked to do.'

Emily said that she was looking forward to being a qualified staff nurse, knowing what she was talking about and able to give realistic, continuous support. Going on to each new ward, she said, was nerve-racking, because you didn't know your way around or how to fit into the team; the temptation was 'to think, Ah, I can do bedpans! and revert back to being task-oriented'. On the whole, however, Emily seemed to be enjoying the process of putting theory into action and making it work. I had the impression that, having begun the course with only vague expectations as to its theoretical side, she was now intellectually engaged and blossoming.

I MET TIM RUSSELL in the pub, the Malt and Hops on St Alphege's Square, much patronized by the hospital staff. It is the usual kind of small city pub, a place of brass rails and rustic-style tables, etched windows and complicated juke boxes. We met in the early evening when it was relatively quiet.

At thirty-four, Tim was the oldest of the student group. At first sight he looked younger, an impression conveyed mainly by his hair – thick, red and cut shaggily – and his clothes: old black jeans and a jumper. Once we had sat down I could see that his face bore all the marks of experience you would expect in a thirty-four-year-old, and yet still the impression of youth persisted. As we talked I realized that, having become used to a certain kind of bouncy, thirty-something male doctor at Alf's, I had been expecting someone similar. The reflectiveness was what had thrown me.

Tim was born and brought up in Dundee, had studied English at university ('only because I couldn't think what else to do') and then worked in retail and, for several years, as the representative of travel companies in southern Europe. He had family in medicine – two sisters were nurses, one was a biologist, yet another was a doctor – so he was fairly well versed in what the job meant when he finally applied to do nursing training.

'I'd heard about Project 2000 vaguely but I only found out at the interview that they were running it at Alf's. I was glad – it's better to have a diploma, which is recognized by universities, than the old RGN certificate. And I wanted to be in on Project 2000 from the start, so that I wouldn't have to retrain later. I considered the mental health branch, but I had no experience in working with mentally ill people and I didn't know if I'd be able to cope. You'd have to be able to leave the work behind when you went home and I've never been good at that.' So Tim signed up for the adult branch.

He had found the CFP 'rather odd. The first six months was very light on work, then suddenly exams hit you. The work could be spread out more evenly. At times there was major stress and everyone was falling out with each other.'

Moreover, on their first placement, he had been keenly aware that the Project 2000 students were anomalies. 'The staff didn't know what to make of us and we had had no preparation for the practical side at all. We didn't even know what a bedpan looked like.'

When Tim and I met, it was December, the CFP was behind him and he had already completed a couple of placements on the branch programme. The Project 2000 students were no longer such strange phenomena to the regular ward staff and Tim found that they were usually welcomed, 'so long as you show you're willing to help. We are still supposed to be supernumerary, and in theory we should be able to say what we want to do, but you don't want to set yourself apart so if you're asked to do something on a busy ward, you do it.'

Tim's long-term future plans were pretty fluid. He liked the idea of going abroad for a few years, perhaps to work with the Red Cross in areas of conflict. For this, a specialization in accident and emergency would be useful. Or he *might* do an extra eighteen months' mental health training after he qualified, to become a Registered Mental Nurse (RMN). There had been a couple of mental health placements on the CFP, which he had found interesting. Going on to do a degree was another option; becoming a practice nurse eventually was yet another.

He was quite clear about the fact that he was looking for a career as well as a vocation. He was now on a placement in the community, working with a practice nurse. (This is a nurse attached to a GP's surgery: the nurse not only assists the doctor but operates autonomously, running special clinics and providing a certain amount of health education. The number of practice nurses is set to multiply as part of the NHS move into the community.)

He said, with a touch of awkwardness, that promotion prospects were good for men in nursing, a fact that was undoubtedly unfair, but gave him encouragement. I asked him if being a man had created any problems for him with other staff or patients. He said no, quite the reverse: 'Studies show that women patients tend to recover faster on wards with a male member of staff. One of my placements has been on a women's stoma ward, which is where people have part of their bowel removed and they get fitted with a stoma, a kind of flesh tube, and a bag. It's a traumatic operation and it's quite damaging psychologically – it gives people problems with their body image. All the nurses on the ward commented that when there was a male member of staff around, the women would get up earlier and make more effort with their hair and make-up. It's probably subconscious but it's good for morale. I spent quite a lot of time talking to those patients; I talked to them as women rather than medical cases and they seemed to enjoy it.'

He liked the autonomy of the job. Being older and of independent mind, he had already come across some aspects of hospital work he didn't like: 'Some wards do things just for the sake of tradition and no one's ever questioned it. Getting everyone up and dressed and in their chairs by 10 o'clock for instance. Sometimes I've asked why and been told it's because we're short-staffed today and it's the only way we can cope, and that's fair enough. But sometimes there is no reason. I'm not sure I could work on a hospital ward like that. Petty rules annoy me, to the extent that I'll break them.'

Tim was also irritated by the way the college seemed to regard students as children. 'For instance, we have to sign an attendance register for lectures. I don't think that's right; we're training for a responsible job. I think you should treat people as adults . . .'

This reminded me of Angela. Perhaps it wasn't surprising that they shared an exasperation at the system, both being older and used to their independence. All the same, I was surprised to discover that Tim was Angela's deputy on the Student Representative Council. He didn't strike me as a committee person at all.

NICOLA DARKE was on the mental health branch and loving it. On the telephone she had sounded clever and considered; she had the soft-spokenness of someone who knew her mind. She was twenty-seven, she had told me, with a degree. Turning up on the appointed evening, at Alf's main gate, I looked around for a face to fit the impression. A small, fair girl was sitting on the bench: she had bobbed hair and a young person's bloom on her cheeks. She looked absolutely nothing like my preconception.

Nicola had always been interested in nursing but her school had considered it insufficiently challenging for her. Following her teachers' advice, she had gone to Oxford, read modern languages and ended up in a job as a technical translator which she hated: 'Sitting in front of a word processor with a pile of books and papers.' After two years at this, she had determined to leave and began investigating her options, including nursing.

She had already developed an interest in mental health and illness. When she'd gone to Europe as part of her degree course she had bypassed the teaching job selected for her and worked with mentally handicapped people instead. Back in the UK, she had trained and worked as a Samaritan. Like Tim and Angela, she had reservations about being able to fit in to the nursing hierarchy, but she was encouraged by what she read of mental health nursing: it seemed to offer a good deal of autonomy and team work.

Nicola was brought up in the Midlands; her translating job had been in Berkshire. She applied to St Alphege's partly for personal reasons – David, her long-term boyfriend, was training to be a solicitor in London – and partly because of Project 2000. She knew that she would be a pioneer on two counts: Project 2000 was brand new here and so was basic training for mental health nursing. The district employs psychiatric nurses on hospital wards and in the community, but up until 1991 St Alphege's offered only post-registration courses in the speciality.

Of all the students, Nicola was the most decided about her future. She was enjoying the course (now that she was on the mental health branch; the CFP had been 'not brilliant') and her placements to date had convinced her that this was what she wanted to do. 'Mental health nursing is intellectually challenging, which I like. It makes you question the things you take for granted about society and people. What makes people tick; why some cope and survive and some don't; what role families play in socialization.'

Her observations on the wards and in the community were already leading her towards a relativist approach: 'To me, while there are some extreme cases of mental illness, people who've lost touch with reality, much of it is an exacerbated version of what all of us feel some of the time – depression, stress. Sometimes personal relationships exacerbate the initial problem; sometimes social conditions do it – in particular bad housing.

'Even in the extreme cases, I don't like to use labels. We do use them, but they're really only shorthand. You say "psychotic" for someone who's lost touch with reality; "schizophrenic" to me would mean someone who's lost touch and who might be hearing voices or seeing things that aren't there, who perhaps feels watched. But beyond that, the terms don't really help. There's a move away from using them now, which I think is quite right.'

Nicola's placements had so far been fairly evenly spread between Alf's, St Wenceslas and the community (for which read the area covered by the St Alphege's and Wavetree District Health Authority). There was limited need for mental health nurses in the commercial district surrounding St Alphege's Hospital, but Wavetree was a largely residential district with high unemployment and severe housing problems, officially acknowledged as one of the poorest boroughs in England. Here there were far more patients than could be catered for on the wards or by community psychiatric teams.

Work often went on in depressing conditions; coping with that was acknowledged to be part of the training. Nicola considered herself lucky to have had a part-time placement on an acute psychiatric ward in St Wenceslas, while she was still on the CFP. 'I thought if I could cope with that, I'd cope with anything. And actually, although the surroundings were awful, it was very interesting and not as threatening as I'd feared.'

On the whole, though, her impressions of St Wenceslas were grim: 'Physically it's a very miserable place, with no money and no facilities. The nurses do the best they can but a lot of them get demoralized. They're the ones who spend most of the shift in the office, doing as little as they can get away with. The worst thing is that there aren't the resources to give patients the attention and therapy they need so there's a bit too much reliance on drug treatment.'

When we met, Nicola had just completed a short placement in a day centre for people with dementia. She had expected to hate it, as during the CFP she'd been on an elderly ward in St Wenceslas and found it deeply depressing. But the centre was new and well staffed, with lots of groups and activities available to the patients, and she had been amazed to find herself enjoying it. 'It just shows what you can do. You can't stop people deteriorating physically but you can make the most of what they've got.'

She was due to start a new placement soon at the Grange, a private hospital on a leafy edge of the St Alphege and Wavetree district. She had seen the expensively printed brochure for the Grange and felt torn about it: eagerness to see how mental health nursing was practised in these surroundings conflicted with a sense that she was betraying the NHS by going. 'Of course, there's no reason why mentally ill people should be treated in horrible, depressing surroundings. They should have nice environments like this. But it seems awful that it's only for the people who can afford to buy their way in.'

ALEXANDRA HALL is an infill, a residential hostel for nurses built into a gap in one corner of the St Alphege's site. It is conveniently placed, which is perhaps why 400 rooms have been crammed into six floors. The corridors are narrow, the stairs steep and there is only one tiny wooden lift, known locally as the Coffin.

Rachel Barlow, however, was pleased to be here. She and a few fellow students from the child branch had 'hassled and hassled' to get transferred from their original rooms over at St Wenceslas. 'I hated that place, it was so depressing, and the journey to come here to college every day was awful. We're such a big group that we couldn't all fit on the minibus so if you were a bit late down you were left at the bus stop in the rain, waiting for London Transport.' She and her friends had finally got themselves neighbouring rooms on the sixth floor of Alexandra Hall.

Rachel's room was narrow, the walls brightened with posters, postcards and photos. The bed was minus its legs. By the window was a sink, a kettle, a portable television and a music centre. I called round at 6 o'clock in the evening, when the corridor was lively with people making tea, preparing dinner and generally unwinding. There were several knocks at the door; at other times people just walked in, already talking.

Rachel was twenty-one, talkative, friendly and insecure. She was brought up near Torquay and worked as a nanny in Sussex before she came to Alf's. She had been waiting to come here ever since 1989. She had originally applied for the RGN course and the introduction of Project 2000 had meant a series of delays. It had also given rise to a misunderstanding which landed her on the child branch almost by default: 'When they wrote and told me about Project 2000 and the branches, I thought that if I did the paediatric branch I'd get both a general nursing and a children's nursing qualification. I'd enjoyed nannying and thought it would be really useful to be qualified to work with children in the future, so I thought great, I'll kill two birds with one stone.'

It was only when she arrived at St Alphege's that Rachel discovered her mistake, and by that time it was too late to change. It was hardly an auspicious start. Nor did it get much better; not academically inclined, Rachel was dismayed to discover how much of the CFP was given over to lectures. She was frustrated by the frequent unpunctuality and absences of the lecturers and found many of the classes that did take place disappointing. She had enjoyed her 'obspar' placements, but there hadn't been enough of them: just thirty-five days, and only four of those had been on a children's ward. Rachel had done agency work to try and increase her ward experience; she was still doing it but she was cagey when I asked her questions about it. She wasn't sure whether the college would approve: as with many aspects of the course, official policy seemed vague.

I found Rachel disarming. She was candid about her feelings and they were confused: she liked living in London but she missed her long-standing boyfriend, Robbie, who lived in Birmingham; she hated the way the CFP had been almost all theory, so much book-learning; on the other hand, now that she was on the branch certain theoretical things were beginning to click into place when she saw them in practice and it was very satisfying. She had no confidence in her academic ability ('I'm average all the way, and I've grown up in the shadow of two very clever sisters') and bad at motivating herself to work, yet when she crammed for exams and projects at the last minute it usually paid off. She always dreaded placements but then she often thoroughly enjoyed them . . . and so on.

She was now beginning a series of part-time placements in the community. The child branch had a strong community bias: during the first few months the students went into schools, nurseries and clinics, and did rounds with health visitors to study normal development in 'the healthy child'. Only after that did they move on to the study of children's diseases and disorders. Rachel had just been out with a health visitor; these days every child under school age is assigned a health visitor who carries out physical check ups at different stages and makes a certain number of home visits to make sure all is well there. 'On home visits she sometimes doesn't even introduce me. I usually just sit there like a stuffed melon. It makes me feel such a twit.' But then again: 'On one visit I picked up the baby and for the first time ever I found myself thinking: 'Three months. Should have good muscle tone. Should be able to hold her head up...' and that was a really exciting feeling. The knowledge is in there somewhere, you see, the penny is dropping.'

Rachel sometimes sounds as if she's a maelstrom of conflicting emotions and attitudes, but in fact she just reacts intensely to things. She likes what she likes, hates what she hates. A lot of it comes down to her being very young. She is also bright, funny and, I suspected by the end of that first interview, quite resilient underneath it all.

JANE RIDDINGTON was on the adult branch. She had already seen enough of British nursing to be disenchanted with it. An only child from Lancashire, she had entered nursing training in pursuit of a worthwhile, rewarding career that offered plenty of opportunities for travel. She had chosen Alf's largely on its reputation: she knew Alf's nurses were internationally recognized. 'Nursing will get me round the world, I think.'

By the time I met her (once again in the Malt and Hops), she was certain that it would have to get her round the world: she didn't want to practise nursing in this country. 'I don't like the way they train nurses here, or the system – there's too much hierarchy. And the pay is terrible. I don't care what anyone says, working with people is not rewarding enough to replace a salary you can live on.'

Jane had come down to London at eighteen, after A levels, and worked in a smaller, specialist hospital as a ward clerk. 'It's a very interesting job: you work on a ward doing the filing, the admin, making sure they've got stocks and stores. You get to see a lot of what goes on on the ward and people tend to talk quite openly in front of you.' She found the nurses themselves 'quite snotty' but liked what she saw of the work and decided to train for it herself. She had been accepted by three London teaching hospitals and chose St Alphege's.

Jane struck me as an odd mixture: she had a laid back manner and a tendency to hang her conversation round hippyish articles of faith. 'I don't like to think about age too much,' she said when I asked her if she was at the younger end of the intake. 'I don't think it says anything important about who you are.' This was in keeping with an overall the-personal-is-universal approach to life; brought up a Christian, she had been introduced to Buddhism by a friend and now practised it. 'Buddhists believe that you can't help anybody unless you help yourself first and are in touch with your own feelings. It's a good philosophy, I think, and one that nurses should take on board.'

Yet behind these bland admonitions, Jane was frequently quite het up. She chafed at numerous aspects of her training: the way the students were given little independence within the course; the hierarchy on the wards; the lack of motivation she perceived among some nurses. She said that she sometimes found it quite difficult on the wards: she didn't like the task-oriented approach of the older RGNs; nor the way some nurses didn't talk to patients, even when carrying out procedures on them.

Jane also felt a purely personal unease when it came to getting along with certain of Alf's staff: 'I've been in London now for about three years. It's very multicultural and half the time I don't know where I am. There are a lot of African Caribbean nurses and I find it difficult to relate to them, simply because I don't know anything about their culture. And they do have a different way of approaching people. For instance I know I'm polite and conservative with people until I get to know them a bit more, but it seems they're very open with people from the word go . . . They'll say what they're feeling; if they're angry or pissed off then they'll show it. Which is great in a way but if you can't handle it, it seems like an insult.'

Coming down to London, Jane said, had made her realize 'how many barriers I had'. She had lived in a village in which everyone came from the same (English) background; even now she was most comfortable 'hanging out with people of my own culture'. But she hoped to go and study at a Buddhist institute in Colorado when she qualified and perhaps eventually work with mentally ill people in a Buddhist environment.

With her combination of naïvety and prickly self-awareness, Jane seemed poised for some time-honoured student experiences. I thought it would be interesting to see how she developed during the second half of the course.

CORRINE TURNER was my seventh student and I didn't meet her face to face until some time after the others. Meanwhile, notes and telephone messages had been travelling between us and verbal messages arrived via her colleagues. Yes, Corinne was interested in being in the book, Emily told me; she had seen her on the bus that morning and Corinne had said so. She had meant to ring earlier, it was just that she was doing her midwifery placement and was very busy. Her personality came filtering through these second-hand reports as easygoing, social, someone with plenty going on in her life. Because she spent much of her free time outside the nursing home, none of the other students I met knew her very well; but then, they all seemed to know her a little. Even Jane, contemplating her 'barriers', said that Corinne was one of the few African Caribbean students she knew to talk to.

I finally met Corinne in her room in St Wenceslas on a sunny afternoon. She was listening to music and pottering; the window was open, letting in birdsong, and there was a comfortable atmosphere in her little room – it seemed more an expression of her personality and less a part of the hostel than the rooms of most students.

Corinne was twenty-three and had been born and brought up in Sheffield. When she was in the sixth form she'd decided to go into nursing and had done a pre-nursing course at a college of further education. 'It was very basic nursing we did there, so we could follow on into RGN training. Two months after it was over, our family moved to London. I wanted some time to settle in to London and do a bit of socializing, so I didn't apply straight away to colleges of nursing. Instead I got a job as a dental nurse. I only meant to do it for a short time but the first six or seven months were really interesting, as I was learning new things, so I stayed on. After a while it became repetitive, though – you weren't really going anywhere after you qualified as a dental nurse. So after about two years I left and applied to St Alf's.'

Like most students, Corinne 'didn't have a clue' about Project 2000 until Alf's wrote and told her. She was happy to do it; her long-term ambition was to be a midwife so she opted for the adult branch.

When I asked what had attracted her to midwifery, Corinne gave a more instinctive answer than Angela had done. She didn't have a strong preference for working with well people rather than sick people, nor was she exercised by considerations of the midwives' autonomy: 'The only thing I'd seen of midwifery then was on the telly but I had a feeling that it was something I'd like to do, to deliver babies. A close friend of my mum's was a midwife and she used to tell me the ups and downs of it, but I was never put off. It is quite an emotional decision to do midwifery, almost a gut feeling.'

She was on her midwifery placement at the moment, working at Wavetree Hospital, and it was living up to expectations. 'I've seen several births now. It's a lovely feeling, just being there. The first time, I didn't think "Eee, it's all horrible" or anything. It was really emotional – it's the only time nursing has actually brought tears to my eyes. The father was there, it was a forceps delivery; they tried the sucker thing at first but the mother just couldn't expel the baby so they used the forceps. That was quite scary, with the tugging and everything. It was a long labour but afterwards, seeing her on the ward all settled was great.'

So far, Corinne said, she was really enjoying the course. (She didn't even mention the CFP, which I confess came as rather a relief.) Now that they were on the wards, time was flying by. She said that she was aware of having an awful lot to learn in the time that remained: she was struck by the confidence of the third-year RGN student nurses she came across on the wards and their high level of practical knowledge. But she found the ward staff were helpful, and so far they had been willing to grant a number of her requests as to where she'd like to work and particular procedures she'd like to learn.

Of all the seven students, Corinne seemed the most independent of hospital life. Her family lived reasonably near by and when she was off duty she tended to mix more with them and with outside friends than with her fellow students. In fact, she appeared not to regard herself as a student in quite the way the others did. I noticed that throughout our first meeting she didn't use the term once. As far as Corinne was concerned, she and her colleagues were nurses, trainee nurses, it was true, and with a few mountains to climb before they registered, but nevertheless, very definitely nurses.

It was obvious that so far Corinne had taken to the work. She talked about it vividly but with a slight shyness; she didn't want to put herself forward as an authority. And on the ward, she said, she sometimes found it difficult to brief doctors about patients: the right words didn't always come when she wanted them. Yet when she talked about her social and family life she was lively and outgoing. It was an interesting contrast and I looked forward to seeing how she worked with patients and fellow nurses on the wards.

The Year Ahead

ALL SEVEN OF these nurses were at the same stage of the course: just getting started on the branch programme, with most of the lectures behind them and a series of placements on wards and in community teams to come. During the year ahead, they would be involved in many kinds of nursing care, in different specialities and under varying conditions.

During the winter months, they would continue to be supernumerary on the wards. They would not be included in staffing numbers and (in theory at least) would not be relied upon to undertake essential nursing care. Their shifts would usually be shorter than the normal eight-hour daytime shifts and they would not do nights. The pattern of two or three days placement work a week, interspersed with college days, would hold good.

In April, they would start their 'rostered service', during which they would be treated as regular staff. They would continue to work on placements (each one lasting between five and ten weeks), but while they were on each ward they would be counted in as a regular member of staff and put on the duty roster for shifts. (Nursing shifts are divided into 'early' about 7 a.m. to 3 p.m.; 'late': about 1.30 p.m. to 9.30 p.m.; and 'night': about 9 p.m. to 8 a.m. Exact start and finish times vary from hospital to hospital and, in Alf's, from ward to ward. The overlap allows for 'handover', when the outgoing nurses brief the incoming ones on the patients.) The students were not yet sure whether they would be expected to do nights on rostered service, but they knew they would be expected to do up to ten days' shifts in a row.

They would be assigned patients to look after and would have regular duties to fulfil. At this stage they would become well and truly part of hospital life.

Rostered duty was due to run from April to October, after which they would be supernumerary again. As part of the training, the students would be assessed on their placement work. They would also have a number of projects to submit and exams to sit. Failure of an exam or a crucial project would entail a resit; a repeated failure would mean they were off the course, barring exceptional circumstances.

The year would end with an elective: a placement which each student would be able to choose. Then more rostered service until the following March – a distant and hazy time from where the students now stood – when those who had stayed the course would finally become registered nurses.

From now until then, I would be tracking the progress of these seven students, learning some of what they learnt, and watching how they coped.

I WOULD ALSO be following five qualified nurses, who were now at work in different parts of the St Alphege's group. Some of them would be crossing paths with the students during the year. Some would be seeing their careers develop in unexpected ways. We shall be meeting them one at a time in the course of the book. Meanwhile, this is what they were doing at the turn of the year.

Sister Janet Moore was in Casualty, where she had been for the last five years. Three years earlier she had been made overall senior sister of the department (full title: Clinical Nurse Manager, Accident & Emergency) and in this role she was in charge of Casualty and Rupert French Ward, a sixteen-bed ward where the emergency admissions went. At thirty-four she was young to have so much senior experience.

Sister Liz Howlett was in the new, well-equipped Marlowe

Ward for AIDS and HIV. Most of the patients had been in for several weeks, fighting one or another of the opportunistic infections which are associated with AIDS. Marlowe Ward was supposed to be the first phase in in-patient treatment of AIDS at Alf's. It was linked to a day clinic and there were plans for expansion. Meanwhile the ward was full, as it almost always was. Two patients were due to go home in the next few days, and staff were busy teaching them how to administer their own medication through surgically implanted tubes. Their beds would be taken immediately by two more waiting to come in.

Staff Nurse Catherine Ford was on Wilcox, the acute psychiatric ward. She had been working there for nearly two years. Patients were referred to Wilcox by their GPs or from community units such as day centres or therapy groups. They came when they could not cope with life outside any more, and their treatment was usually a mixture of medication, psychotherapy (given by trained therapists) and skilled psychiatric nursing.

The nursing, as provided by Catherine and her colleagues, involved a good deal of one-to-one interaction. The nature of the work changed according to the type of patients on the ward at any one time: they might be diagnosed as schizophrenic, with violent behavioural problems and long-term reliance on drugs. They might be depressive and have attempted suicide. They might have an obsessive compulsive disorder such as repeated handwashing, making it impossible for them to live a normal life. The aim was always to rehabilitate them so that they could move back into the community.

The fourth nurse was over at St Wenceslas: Enrolled Nurse Christine Carton had been twelve years on Hamilton Ward, the long-stay elderly care ward for women. The women on the ward were not strictly speaking sick, but they were old and could not live alone any longer. Most of them had dementia to some degree; many were incontinent. Nursing them was not a matter of working towards a cure, but of trying to give them a decent quality of life.

At fifty, Christine had twenty-four years' experience in nursing. But because she was an enrolled rather than a registered nurse (with one year's less training), she could not be promoted. The senior nurse in charge of elderly care wanted her to do a conversion course and become an RGN: then she could take on the responsibility and get the promotion she deserved. However, it was a two-year course which had to be pursued largely in her own time, and Christine was not inclined to take on such a large commitment at the moment. So far it was proving a busy enough winter and rather a sad one: two of the patients for whom she was a named nurse had died.

The fifth nurse was at the other end of the experience spectrum: Staff Nurse Kate Marshall had just qualified and was preparing for her first day in her first job. It was to be on Howard Ward, a general children's ward in St Alphege's. Kate had done a degree course, specializing in psychology and nursing, so paediatrics was a new departure for her. She was excited and, as the approach of the New Year brought the prospect of her first day, increasingly nervous.

Winter

THE TWO CHILDREN'S wards in St Alphege's, Walsh, a cancer ward and Howard, a general ward, are in the same small block, on the north side of Alf's main courtyard: Walsh is on the first floor, Howard on the second, where it gets the benefit of more daylight.

The fact that Howard is lighter and brighter was one of the things to strike Kate Marshall when she was applying for jobs on both. In retrospect she wondered how much of the impression had been created by other factors: the graver degree of sickness in most of the children on Walsh, for example, and the fact that many of them were strapped up to drips. With only two children's wards in Alf's, she did not have a great deal of choice as to where to work, but she was more attracted to the atmosphere and the range of work on Howard.

As a general ward, Howard admits children from the local district for all kinds of routine complaints. They come in to have their tonsils out, to have teeth extracted, to have asthma monitored. Quite a high percentage of admissions come through Casualty: they may stay in hospital to be treated for burns or broken bones, or to have investigations into symptoms like severe stomach pains.

But Howard Ward also specializes in bowel diseases and children come here from all over the country and sometimes from abroad to receive treatment. As these diseases tend to be long term, the same children return again and again, often for long periods. From a nursing point of view, they present a challenge and an opportunity: the nurses must help them cope with their disease and give them a good quality of life in hospital, without allowing them to become institutionalized.

It was the first days of the New Year and many of the hospital staff were still away on their Christmas break. So were the patients: on Kate's first day only four of the twenty-four beds were occupied; on her second only three were filled. There was plenty of time for what was called her 'orientation': like all new nursing staff, she was to spend several days being shown around the wards and any associated clinics, meeting the people she would work with, being trained on the computer and shown how to use equipment. In fact, there was so much time and so little to do with it that the sister sent her home early on each of her first three days. Next week, she was promised, the real work would begin. Howard Ward would be back to normal, as it had been when she came on her job candidate's visit.

Kate Marshall was twenty-four and came from Shropshire. She was engaged to Paul, a farmer. By background and inclination, she was a country person; in appearance too. She had a rounded figure, very nice skin and soft straight dark hair. At our first meeting I was struck by the absence of that slightly frenetic quality that hangs round most Londoners. Kate seemed grounded and, as the French say, 'happy in her skin'. There was a distinct lack of urban hard edges about her manner. Yet for the last four and a half years she had been leading a very urban life, living in the heart of commercial London, going to lectures amongst the office blocks and working on placement in the wards of Alf's and its associated hospitals.

'Before I came here, I was petrified,' she said. 'My parents hate cities. They were born in Birmingham and moved out at the first opportunity, and I've always lived in the country. I felt that if I could come to London, I could do anything I wanted to. If I could cope with that, I could go anywhere in the world and nothing would be a problem.'

She had enjoyed being in the city, on the whole. It had been a good place to live as a student, 'going to the cinema at 11 o'clock at night and having a choice of what to see. And the theatre. And I used to love walking round the West End.' She had wanted her first job to be here, partly out of sentiment, partly because of the cachet attached to experience at Alf's. Moreover, it made sense to capitalize on the fact that Alf's still offered jobs to its newly trained nurses.

Until very recently, it was taken for granted that nurses were offered jobs by the institution which trained them. So long as you completed the course satisfactorily and became a registered/enrolled/graduate nurse, you could expect to find a job at the same hospital. In many cases, newly qualified nurses could even request a particular ward and have a good chance of being placed there. In the last few years this has changed drastically. Budget cuts have meant fewer vacancies and Kate's was one of the last generations to be able to expect 'home' jobs. She and her colleagues were well aware of this at the time.

The nursing degree students were a small group: eight had begun the course, six of them saw it through to the end. Only a small percentage of British nurses train this way, though the numbers are rising. Most who choose this route do so because they see it as widening their options for the future. All nurses nowadays have to do additional courses of study after they qualify, to prove that they are keeping up to date. A minimum level of continuing study is necessary for nurses to keep their jobs; above that, courses carry credits which help advance their grades and improve their promotion prospects. A degree nurse registers with more academic credits to her name than an RGN; she also has useful experience of independent study. Then again, if she should leave nursing, she can apply for other jobs on the basis of being a graduate.

These considerations had drawn Kate to the degree. The

course offered by Alf's, with the nearby university, was an associated one: each student did nursing classes and placements and specialized in one subject within the social science department. Kate chose psychology.

It was a four-year course. The students spent an initial year working on the wards at Alf's; then they attended the university for three years, tackling a full timetable of lectures and academic work. In the summer holidays they returned to Alf's to do more placement work on the wards. And, just like the Project 2000 students, they all did a certain amount of agency work at Alf's during term-time, to earn extra money.

As the end of their course approached, they all began worrying about jobs. Rumours were circulating about a shortfall and the degree nurses would be qualifying at the same time as a batch of RGNs; there would be about fifty people looking for places.

They had been promised that a list of vacancies would be put up in personnel two weeks before they sat their nursing finals. But in the event the Tomlinson Report was published then, throwing Alf's management into turmoil, and the list did not make its appearance until the day of the exam itself. There were four fewer jobs than nurses; they were each allowed to apply for just two. It was a time of intense pressure and competition.

Kate was interested in midwifery, paediatric nursing and teaching, but found her immediate options limited. She had investigated the possibility of becoming a nursing tutor, but had discovered that it would require not only a degree but a masters and a PhD. She'd had enough study for the time being. She was attracted to the idea of teaching health issues in schools, but jobs in the field are not over-abundant and that too would mean taking further course of study. Midwifery meant another eighteen months' study and in any case she would need six months' experience as a qualified nurse first.

At the time of finals, the best option seemed to be to take a job in one of the areas of nursing which interested her and think again later. Kate and Paul were planning to get married the following September and she would be moving to Shropshire. With Alf's future in doubt and upheaval taking place in almost every quarter of the NHS, it was impossible to say what the situation would be then.

Paediatric nursing attracted on several counts. She could apply for jobs as a junior staff nurse without further study, the experience would stand her in good stead for midwifery and if she decided to continue in the field she could work for a specialist RSCN (Registered Sick Children's Nurse) qualification.

All sick children in hospital have the right to be treated by a registered sick children's nurse. This means that every children's ward must employ at least one RSCN on each shift; it also means that positions of responsibility, such as sisters, can only be filled by RSCNs. A nurse becomes an RSCN in several ways: in pre-Project 2000 days, a three-year RSCN course existed as an alternative to the RGN. For Project 2000 students, there is the option of taking the child branch. And nurses who have qualified as RGNs can take post-registration RSCN courses; this was what Kate might decide to do. She duly submitted two application forms, one to Howard, one to Walsh. 'It was a bit of a farce really – they both had exactly the same information on them, right down to my reasons for wanting that particular job.'

As a job applicant, she was given an informal tour of each ward. While she liked the look of Howard, she was daunted by Walsh. It wasn't just the appearance of the ward: much of the nursing there was oriented around chemotherapy (the administration of strong drugs, mainly intravenously, to control cancer) and seemed very specialized. She was also put off by the fact that the sisters who showed her round seemed under a lot of stress. She opted for Howard as her first choice and was relieved when she was offered the staff nurse vacancy there.

Although Kate's first few days on the ward were something of an anti-climax after all her nervous anticipation, they at least gave her time to familiarize herself with the layout. It was not a traditional open ward: instead the patients were accommodated in four four-bedded bays and four side rooms. At any one time the age range on the ward might be from infancy to eighteen, but as far as possible children were put in with others of the same age and sex. When occupied, the bays and rooms tended to be quite sociable places. There was a television and video in each and many children brought their own videos and computer games with them.

Near the entrance to the ward was a playroom and three other rooms which were used as classrooms. (During term-time teachers came on to the ward every day to help the children keep up their education.) Then there were the usual ward facilities: a linen room, a sluice, a room where all the bits of equipment – drips, tubing, blood pressure belts and so on – were kept, and a staff room.

When Kate came back on duty the next Monday, after a weekend off, the ward was transformed. New patients were arriving with their parents and the playroom was full of children waiting to be admitted. The staff were unfamiliar – those she had been on duty with last week were now taking time off – and too busy to be gentle with her. 'It was "Well, you've had your orientation: do this, that and the other!" '

One of her first tasks was to admit an eight-year old girl who had come in for treatment of Crohn's Disease. Admitting patients is an important part of nursing: it involves taking a medical history of the patient and noting down extensive information about their personal health and circumstances. There are admissions forms with standard questions to be completed. But the nurse also has to be alert enough to pick up other signals: skin and hair in poor condition might be a sign of malnutrition, for instance.

Admitting children usually means dealing with the child and the parents (or other carers) together. The questions may have to be asked of everyone in turn; parents and children may require differing degrees of explanation as to what is going to happen. An RSCN will have undergone special training in how to talk to children about their illnesses; Kate had to rely on her instincts and her observations of how the other staff were proceeding.

The history that emerged of Emma Poole was a gruelling one, for Emma had suffered from Crohn's Disease since infancy. Crohn's is a particularly nasty disorder which produces ulcers in the digestive system, occuring anywhere between the mouth and the anus, very often in the bowel. These ulcers are extremely painful; their cause is unknown and no permanent cure has yet been developed. Adults and children can both get Crohn's, and the disease can be debilitating whatever the age of the patient. Children with severe Crohn's often find it very difficult to live a normal life. They may have to have twenty or thirty bowel movements a day, each excruciatingly painful. Their digestion no longer functions properly; in addition they lose their appetite. This incurs the risk of them not growing properly, quite apart from the loss of all the usual childhood activities.

Howard Ward at St Alphege's is an internationally known specialist centre for the treatment of Crohn's. Emma had been a patient there for years, coming in for courses of treatment which often lasted weeks at a time. She'd had steroid treatment, which had worked temporarily, and several operations to remove ulcerated sections of her bowel. Some time before, she had had a colostomy, a procedure in which the colon is removed and the end of the intestine is brought to the surface of the abdomen via a 'stoma', a surgically created tube of flesh.

Unfortunately, ulcers had now occurred elsewhere in her bowel. She was passing blood and mucus when she went to the toilet and was very anaemic. She was in pain and distress for much of the time. Over previous months she had managed to get her school attendance up to two mornings a week, but now she couldn't even walk to the corner shop because the urge to have a bowel movement would overwhelm her several times en route.

Severe as Emma's condition was, she was an old hand at hospital life and quite unfazed by being readmitted. Howard Ward was a second home to her and she knew how everything worked. Kate found her rather daunting.

'Why are you getting that bed ready, Katherine?' Emma asked, reading the name on Kate's badge. 'I want this bed here. I always have it.' She then proceeded to veto the proposed duvet cover and select another. As Kate continued to try and settle her in and chat to her, she took exception to several of her questions. No one, she informed Kate loftily, had ever asked her that before.

By the end of the day, Kate was feeling something close to dislike for the child. She felt guilty about the reaction, but it was hard to take to such an imperious little person. Emma knew the normal routine, what time meals were served; she was used to who did which tasks and how. These were all things which Kate was having to learn as she went. Meanwhile Emma demanded to know why 'Katherine' hadn't brought her her medicine yet, and why wasn't her favourite book by her bed?

The temptation to leave Emma's nursing to others was strong. Kate had her work cut out as it was, getting to know the ward, the other patients and the staff. One nurse in particular seemed inclined to be snappish and had already given Kate a few sharp remarks.

'But when I thought about it, I realized how institutionalized Emma was. She was probably typical of quite a few children who were going to be on the ward – Crohn's is our specialism and children who suffer from it come in again and again. So I thought I'd better learn to deal with it. And I also thought that if I could make friends with *Emma*, I was made. She'd make my life so easy and look out for me in a way, because if I did anything wrong she'd say straight away, "Oh you shouldn't be doing it like that!" '

So Kate set about trying to win Emma's confidence. It wasn't easy: for Emma, the ward really was an alternative home, where she knew the staff and had well-established relationships. A newcomer on the scene was difficult for her to cope with. But Kate persevered, spending time talking to Emma and playing with her. During the next few days they played Scrabble and Cluedo. They read stories. They made friendship bracelets. Kate made sure that she was around to help with Emma's routine care: getting her up and dressed, helping her wash, giving her the special nutritious liquid she had been prescribed instead of food in order to rest her digestive system. Meanwhile, of course, Emma was only one child on a ward that had now swelled to twelve, and Kate found that the settling in process involved learning to operate at a number of different speeds.

Howard Ward almost always has a few regulars like Emma on it, children with long-term illnesses, who make repeated visits of several weeks at a time to have their treatment updated or adjusted. These are usually, but not always, children with bowel disease. Other children might be in with a one-off acute illness like jaundice; or for treatment of a chronic condition such as asthma or hormone imbalance. They might be staying in only a night or two for routine surgery, the removal of tonsils or adenoids, for instance; or they might be in for major surgery such as a heart operation.

To be a nurse on a children's ward like this requires a good deal of flexibility. It also requires stamina. For sick children do not necessarily behave as if they are sick – once their pain is relieved, their greatest bugbear is boredom. On Howard it is recognized that the children will probably not want to stay in bed and the ward is arranged and days structured to give them plenty of things to do.

There are three teachers on Howard; they give lessons on weekdays from 9.30 a.m. to 12 and from 2 till 3.30 p.m. Children are divided up by age for the lessons, which are known on the ward as 'school'. It is not much like a formal school, however; lessons tend to be imaginative and activity based, with much making of things like compasses and pinhole cameras.

All children over the age of five are expected to attend school unless they are feeling ill, in which case they must explain the fact to the teachers. If they are too ill to get up but well enough to do some work, the teachers give them work to do in bed. Mostly, the children like it, as it gives them something to do. The treasured Nintendo is out of bounds during the day and televisions have to stay turned off.

The nurses carry on their work amidst this constant activity. The New Year period was a busy one, with plenty of new admissions. Children with bowel disease who had been at home for Christmas were coming back in for more treatment. This often meant putting them on to a liquid diet, like Emma's, and administering steroids in enema or injection form. Then there were spates of surgery.

Operations such as tonsilectomies, the removal of adenoids and putting grommets in ears are scheduled to come in batches, so that the surgical team in the theatre gets a straight run at them. That year, St Alphege's had contracts with a number of GPs to provide tonsilectomies and Howard was experiencing regular 'tonsilectomy days', when up to six children might be operated on. This made for a lot of work on the ward. The children all needed to be admitted the day before, prepared for general anaesthetic by having their food and water intake stopped, accompanied to and from theatre on the day itself and given after care once the operation was over.

Under these circumstances, the ideal approach to preparing a child for an operation – 'getting on the floor and playing with the child and explaining to them what's going to happen', as Kate put it – comes under pressure. On a day when half a dozen children are going for surgery, all the nurses on the ward tend to be working at full pelt. Each nurse develops her own personal way of imparting information plainly and swiftly, and grows skilled at anticipating anxieties.

'You always try to explain to children *and* to the parents. For instance, the parents can come to the anaesthetic room and watch the child being put to sleep. They can come to recovery when the child is waking up. The only bit they don't see is in between. So parents often need counselling as they don't know what to expect. If they've ever had an operation, they've generally been too sleepy to remember. Or they might have had a bad experience themselves.

'If you have a five- or six-year-old child who's going to have its tonsils out, you go through what is going to happen and make sure Mum and Dad are there listening as well. Then you have to check out the child's understanding of what's going to happen. Then you have a quiet word with Mum and Dad and ask if there's anything else that needs explaining. Generally, you've had to make it so simple for the children that most parents are quite happy with it.'

While Kate hadn't received the specific training in communicating with children which the RSCN course would have given her, her psychology degree had included clinical and health psychology and developmental psychology. She had therefore studied how much children can understand at different ages. She had also looked at social and physical aspects of childhood, an area of study covering what children understand, how they behave and how to explain things to them.

On tonsilectomy days the ward is crowded with patients and parents. On Howard, parents are actively encouraged to stay with their child. Alf's can offer them accommodation in Surgery House, a separate building near the two children's wards, built and run with charity money; its rooms have been furnished by one of the big chain stores and it is equipped with bathrooms and a kitchen. Parents and other family members can stay here while a child is on the wards. It's a particularly useful facility for families from other parts of the country whose children have been referred on to Alf's (often for Crohn's or other bowel diseases). If Surgery House is full, parents who want to stay overnight with their children are given a comfortable chair by the bed. If their child is in a bay and the next door bed is empty, parents are allowed to put a sheet over the duvet and sleep there – though they might well be asked to get up in the night if the bed is needed.

All in all, parents, especially mothers, are a permanent feature of life on Howard Ward. They carry out a good deal of the routine care of their own children, washing and feeding them, helping them in and out of bed, taking them to the toilet. On busy theatre days, when Kate seemed to spend all her time running up and down to theatres and pre- and post-operation observations placed a heavy burden on the staff, she noticed that the parents would often step in to deal with any minor upsets, crossing the ward to comfort a crying child, or taking restless ones into the playroom to organize a game.

The care of tonsilectomy patients after their operations is straightforward: the children are kept in overnight, under observation, and the next morning they are given something crunchy to eat – toast or cornflakes or, if they prefer, crisps. The process of swallowing the crunchy food cleans the tonsil bed, scouring off any bits of scab or dried blood and helping to prevent infection. Once the children have eaten, they are allowed to leave, with instructions to their parents that they must go on eating something crunchy each day for several days.

In theory, it's simple, but Kate quickly discovered the catch: getting children to eat the post-tonsilectomy breakfast can be murder. 'Oh, it's awful. They all sit there with their cornflakes or Rice Krispies or toast, and they're not feeling bad at this stage. You've given them some medicine before and they've swallowed that all right. They take a big mouthful because they're hungry and then half way down they realize it's going to hurt. And it does – I tried doing it last week when I had tonsilitis and it was *so* painful! But they have to eat it or they end up with a scab on the tonsil bed which just grows and gets infected. So then you're standing there saying, "You can't go home till you've eaten that whole piece of toast. Yes, all of it. And the crust!" And they're staring at you in outrage.'

With younger children, she found, she could usually get a result by being authoritarian – 'You've *got* to eat it!' – or by presenting it as something slightly naughty – 'This is your excuse to have a packet of crisps every single day!' But older children, and especially adolescents, would resist for hours.

In Kate's third week, two fourteen-year-olds were admitted on the same day for tonsilectomy. They were big, strapping lads: both of them did weight training; they had each come in with a handful of '18' horror and cop videos. They were men, not boys, they told the nurses repeatedly, as they watched the videos together and swapped muscle-bound anecdotes. The next morning they were sitting up in bed in a bay with a three-year-old who had had a multiple procedure – adenoids and tonsils out and grommets put in his ears. And Kate, doing the toast-for-breakfast routine, was not especially surprised to find herself faced with two fourteen-year-old men squeaking in pained outrage while the three-year-old munched his way stoically through his toast.

'They were sat there saying, "But it *hu-urts*! You can't make me do that! It *hu-urts*!" And there was this little chap who'd had everything done to him eating away. I said, "Look at him, he's bigger than the pair of you. Are you mice or men?" "I think we're mi-i-i-ce!" And all the time there was *Pet Semetary* by Stephen King playing away on the video.'

Nor is it always simple to make parents understand the necessity of the crunchy food regime. Briefing the parents of an eight-year-old who'd had to be kept in an extra six hours before he'd eat some crisps, Kate had an uneasy sensation that she wasn't getting through. No matter how many times she explained exactly why he had to be made to eat crunchy food over the next week, the parents continued to protest that surely it wasn't kind when his throat hurt. Kate saw them go home with misgivings. Sure enough, seven days later the boy was back, his throat so badly infected that he was dribbling. (The treatment was predictable: antibiotics for the infection and more of the dreaded crunchy things to eat.)

After several weeks on Howard, Kate was beginning to take stock of just what was involved in paediatric nursing. 'It's very different from nursing adults because parents tend to carry out the care of the child. On Howard, for instance, you're very rarely washing a child. So the work is less physically demanding. Mentally, it's much harder because the children need to be occupied and they have so much energy. They're usually running around everywhere and you've got to be constantly watching to make sure they can't get hold of anything sharp or dangerous. You have to be so much more of a bully – I feel like I'm more of a school teacher every day.

'Children are so straightforward, that's what I like. It hurts or it doesn't. They're ill or they're not. They like you or they don't. With an adult it's, "Well, it sort of hurts . . ." A child doesn't know, for instance, if it's going to be sick. It just is, and you deal with it.

'Also, children are much more independent than adult patients. Adults tend to say, "Just sit me up in bed, nurse," and two of you do it and it's fine. With children it's, "No, no, I want to do it myself." We have children here who've just had really big bowel operations, with tubes and wires everywhere, and they're determined to get themselves sitting up in bed. You have to respect that. But you also need to help them, because of all the wires and tubes, and to see that they don't damage the wound. It can take half an hour for a child to get sat up and comfortable; it would have taken you two minutes.'

In some ways, sick children's nursing is a more nebulous discipline than adult nursing: nurses spend a good deal of their time providing comfort, encouragement and information rather than carrying out specific procedures. At the end of a month, Kate already perceived an overlap here with health promotion: she was looking into the possibility of formalizing it by putting up a health promotion noticeboard on the ward. 'I think we could address a different issue every two weeks, with a display of leaflets and posters: smoking; dental hygiene; alcohol. It would be useful for the parents as much as the children.'

Yet where medicalized procedures are involved, the care is subject to very strict parameters. Drug administration, for instance, is more complicated with children. 'Checking drugs is always important because the dose must be right. But at least with adults, patients generally get the same dose for the same condition. You get to know that a gram of paracetamol is fine. But with a child, it depends on the body weight: if the child only weighs 20 kilos you wouldn't want to give it a gram of paracetamol. You have to work out the correct dose each time, according to weight.'

Hospital regulations state that all drug administration to children must be supervised by a registered sick children's nurse. As there is an RSCN on each shift, this is perfectly possible, if sometimes tiresome. However, Kate found herself on a drug round with a staff nurse who, although not an RSCN, proceeded to sign the supervision form.

Kate wasn't happy about it. It wasn't that she mistrusted the nurse, who had been on the ward for years, but it had been inculcated into her during her training that accountability was of the first importance; legally the form required the signature of an RSCN. This particular staff nurse was not amenable to that kind of argument. She was not particularly amenable at all – she had been curt with Kate on several previous occasions and Kate had already learnt to be wary of her.

'I said, "Really, you ought not to be signing this. We're not covered if you make a mistake." And she said, "Don't be stupid, I've been here twelve years and I've always done it in the past!" '

The staff nurse signed. Moreover, she had been offended and she showed it by putting Kate through the hoops on the rest of the drug round. 'For one child we were having to add two drugs together. There was a bag of saline [salty water] and we were having to add an antibiotic. It was a ridiculous dose: mix it up with this bit of water and empty it into this bag . . . it was 45 milligrams out of a 1 gram bottle and you had to mix it with 0.8 of a millilitre of water. You had to do the calculations to work it out. And the staff nurse said, "Have you worked it out? How much of this fluid do we have to inject?" And I said, "Well, if it was 50 mg it would be this much, and it's not quite that so it's this." And she said, "No, you've got it wrong."

'Now, I always work things out in my head. She said, "Try again." And I kept trying to work it through to get it to a different answer and she was saying, "Come on! Come on! Faster! You're not safe to give drugs if you can't do this simple calculation. Use the formula!" '

The formula is a simple arithmetical one taught as part

of nursing training. Kate had never had any problem with it before, but now she was flustered. She asked for a moment to do the calculations again, whereupon the staff nurse began impatiently writing out the formula on a paper towel. The answer she reached was the same one Kate had already given. There then followed a tit-for-tat argument.

'I said it was that!'

'No you didn't!'

'Yes I did and you told me it was wrong!'

'Did I? Oh well, I'm sorry, but you must know how to do this. Get yourself a calculator so you know you're always giving the right amount.'

The incident rocked Kate's confidence. She no longer trusted herself to do the calculations correctly, with or without the formula. For all the following week she kept taking drugs to other members of staff and asking them if she'd got the dose right. 'They'd say, "Yes Kate," in a patient sort of way. I was trying to prove to everyone that I could do this calculation and give drugs safely. It's the whole status of the staff nurse – you can do things safely. I felt I had to prove it to the whole world. But nobody was interested except for this one nurse who'd made a mistake in the first place.'

That particular staff nurse, Kate came to realize, was considered by most people to be difficult. She had been working on Howard for twelve years, for most of them as an enrolled nurse. As such, her length of experience had far outstripped the use to which she could put it, enrolled nurses having no promotion prospects and being restricted in the amount of responsibility they can take. She had recently completed a conversion course and was now an RGN, and whether it was because she resented having had to requalify, or because she was trying too hard to prove herself, or simply because she was that kind of person, she always seemed ready for confrontation. Kate dreaded having to ask her anything, as the response was usually a snap. Her attitude to Kate's plan for the health promotion board was 'Well, if you've got nothing better to do with your time . . .'

Realizing that the other staff felt as she did helped Kate not to take this nurse's remarks too personally. Nevertheless, she kept out of her way as much as possible.

On most fronts, meanwhile, Kate was making progress. At the end of the first week, she scored a small but significant triumph: Emma, the little girl with Crohn's Disease, climbed on to her lap and declared that today she would rather be with Kate than anyone else. Singling out one person for approval or dislike was standard behaviour for Emma: the other nurses told Kate that the little girl had long since learnt to manipulate people. She could be especially tricky with her mother. It was one of the only ways in which Emma could exercise independence – she had been suffering bouts of agonizing pain since she was tiny; she was very often off school and had to endure long periods in hospital. She relied heavily on her mother, for comfort and stability, and it was her mother who bore the brunt of Emma's frustration.

Emma's treatment at the moment consisted of replacing food with TPN (Total Parental Nutrition, a milky liquid which meets all the body's nutritional needs) and having regular enemas, which would help heal the ulcers in her bowel. Sometimes the nurses gave the enemas; sometimes her mother did. Whenever her mother gave it, Emma insisted that it hurt, yet she had no complaints when it was the nurses' turn. Her mother, naturally, found this very distressing.

The nurses didn't think Emma truly found it painful when her mother gave the enema, they thought it was more likely a mixture of embarrassment and anger. The emotional fall out could be handled on the ward, where the mother could get support from nurses and the other parents, and where the nurses could step in when it got too much. But Emma would need to continue having the drugs after she was discharged and all the staff were worried that the mother wouldn't be able to cope at home. It wasn't feasible to arrange for a district nurse to come in and give the enemas, as she wouldn't be able to spend enough time with Emma to get her to take them calmly. So it was decided, with Emma's doctor, to stop enemas and start her on a new drug which could be given as an injection. Emma's ulcers had been healing well with the enemas; now they had to hope that the new drug would be as successful.

During these early weeks on Howard, Kate's learning curve was formidable. The range of conditions on the ward and the cross-section of ages under her care (from birth to eighteen) meant that she was continually assessing and re-evaluating her approach, patient by patient. She was also amassing clinical information about the children's conditions; for this she found the care plans, which were in every patient's notes, extremely valuable.

On the basis of the information obtained on admission, the nurses draw up a care plan, which identifies the patient's problems and works out how the nursing care will address them. For instance, if a child comes into Howard in pain, one of the care plan's main aims might be to make him pain-free within thirty minutes of complaining of it. The plan then identifies ways of achieving that: positioning him in a more comfortable place; giving him a heat pad; trying distraction therapy. It states how staff will assess the pain; what analgesia they will give; how they are going to monitor it. The care plan is then evaluated each day, to see how far these aims have been achieved.

By reading the care plans and asking senior staff anything she was still unsure of, Kate found that her knowledge was increasing in leaps. All the same, there were occasions almost every day when she felt that she would never catch up with the others. And the work was tiring.

Officially, nurses are allowed to work ten days in a row without a break, but most wards try to avoid asking staff to do this. The sister on Howard aimed to keep stretches of duty down to eight days at the most, because at the end of that nurses tended to be tired and short-tempered and unable to cope well with the children.

Kate had been given day shifts up till now, so she didn't have to cope with the disorientation of night duty, but when February arrived she was still pretty tired. She had three days off duty coming up. She added two days of her annual leave entitlement to them and made arrangements to go up to Shropshire. She had a craving to breathe some clean air and walk around the garden without having to look out for broken glass. She also wanted to see Paul, her fiancé. They had been going out for almost six years now. When Kate had come to London they had made no promises to each other; they'd both thought it more than likely that they would drift apart. But the opposite had happened and in Kate's last year at university they had got engaged. The wedding was set for September and they were having a new house built for themselves on Paul's family farm. Kate took herself off to Shropshire with a long list of things to do.

THE STUDENT on the child branch, Rachel Barlow, had meanwhile been studying 'the healthy child'. Her January had been very different from Kate's: while Kate worked on the ward, getting to grips with the practicalities of caring for sick children, Rachel was visiting schools.

The child branch syllabus had already devoted November and December to the study of healthy nought- to five-year-olds. Now it was sending the students out to observe six- to sixteen-year-olds in the community. The idea behind this was that in order to learn about ill health and disorders in children, the students should first become familiar with what is defined as normal development.

Before Christmas, Rachel and the others in the group had

been going on rounds with health visitors – those sometimes interesting, sometimes uncomfortable sessions during which Rachel would, as she put it, 'sit there like a stuffed melon'. She had also visited a nursery school and a reception class (for four- to five-year-olds) in a primary school. January saw her back in the same primary school, concentrating on six- to eleven-year-olds.

Rachel had not been impressed by the placement. The amount of time she spent in the school was limited to three days, when she was attached to the school nurse. School nurses are based in health centres and are assigned a list of schools to visit. They help doctors carry out medical tests; they do a certain amount of health education; they carry out check ups and liaise with parents when necessary.

To Rachel, the job seemed indeterminate and not particularly rewarding: 'Well, when I went visiting with the nurse, I got very good at filing. I looked at some nits. We did primary school medicals for five-year-olds – a doctor has to be there and the nurse aids the doctor. I only spent the three days with her and most of it was me sitting in her office, waiting for her to turn up.'

Rachel was also seriously fed up with the academic side of the course. She felt that too much time was being spent on the healthy child; she was worried about how they wouldn't be able to cover all the necessary aspects of caring for sick children, when the course eventually got round to it. But most galling was the fact that the lecturers were unreliable: very often they were late for their own lectures and sometimes they didn't turn up at all.

'We're expected to hang round for half an hour, before we leave, otherwise we get put down as not having attended! So we can wait half an hour for a lecture that's supposed to be one hour long, and then we'll go to the college office and find that there's a message that the tutor's sick, or has cancelled the lecture, but no one's bothered to pass it on to us. So then we've got to do that work in our own time, and our reading lists are huge anyway.'

Some weeks, half of the lectures were cancelled or started late. All the students in the set were annoyed about it and complained to the college. Rachel was the branch's representative on the Student Council and she was thinking about raising the matter at the next meeting.

Between vanishing lectures and placements spent filing, Rachel wasn't feeling very pleased with the course. The part of it she was enjoying was contact with children, when she could get it. She had managed to get some at the primary school, when she was released from the school nurse's office and given permission to go round the classes and chat to the pupils. It was an inner city school, in a tough part of the Wavetree borough, and she expected that after school the children would be playing football in the parks, or roller skating in the streets, or getting up to some kind of imaginative (and possibly destructive) do-it-yourself game. What she found surprised her.

'Among the ten-year-olds virtually every child I spoke to had a computer and would go home and play on the Sega Megadrive. I wasn't taken aback that they knew how to use them, but that they all *had* them. They're living in Wavetree and they're ten years old and they've all got hi-fis and televisions in their rooms. That amazed me. I said, "Don't you hang out with your bicycles, or on your roller boots?" And they said, "Well, sometimes," but they've all got mountain bikes.

'There were three boys – the real lads of the year, they were smashing – and they all go over to each other's houses at weekends and stay up till 2, 3, 4 o'clock in the morning trying to finish the computer game. I don't really know what boys do at that age (I didn't have any brothers), but I was still playing with my Sindy or my pogo stick, or netball with my sister.'

In the second half of January, she had a placement at a secondary school. Feeling nervous about going to an inner city secondary, she decided to make use of contacts and called her sister, who taught at a secondary school in a west London suburb. She managed to get herself invited on placement there, the college agreed to it and here, at last, sitting in on lessons at every stage throughout the school, she thoroughly enjoyed herself.

'It was really, really amusing watching the adolescents. It was exactly like when I was at school – there was always a group of goody-goodies, squares; they were always boys, wearing their blazers. Then there was a group of girls who were really good and getting on with their work. Then there was a group of girls who were testing the water and chatting the boys up – they had their make-up on and the earrings and the hair. And then there was the lads. It hasn't changed at all! I could've watched them all day, it was so funny.'

Rachel had always liked adolescents, she said; she was touched by their fledgling status: – almost but not quite adults, just beginning to see the world open up before them.

This school visit, like the other, lasted only a few days, then Rachel was back in college. At the start of February, though, she had another, more harrowing encounter. It was a Saturday night and Rachel was doing one of her occasional agency night shifts. ('I never look forward to it – it's bedpans, bed baths, dogsbody stuff. I do it for the money, but actually once I'm there, I enjoy it.') She reported for duty on Preston, an adult cancer ward. They were having a heavy night as they had several patients who were very ill and suffering badly. One of the sickest of these turned out to be very young, a boy still in his teens. Rachel listened to his history at handover and then quietly asked the other nurses about him. She discovered that he had been diagnosed with leukaemia at ten. He had been given treatment and the cancer had gone into remission; he'd got better and had been able to return to school. But then the cancer returned, more widespread, and now he was terribly ill.

Rachel was very shaken by what she saw that night. 'His kidneys had packed up, his liver had packed up – he was having massive blood transfusions and as it went in it was clotting. He was vomiting blood. His hair was coming out; his fingernails were dead. You just looked at him and little parts of him were dying.'

The physical symptoms were distressing in themselves, but what really affected her was the sense of the boy's lost future. 'It's probably because I haven't been in contact with it very much, but it seems to me that when they're *very* young, although it's tragic if they're going to die, they haven't known much of what the future could hold anyway. But when they're older, they realize what they're losing. And sixteen, seventeen, that's such an important age. Your toes are on the edge. You've just got it all ahead of you.'

Rachel came off duty on the Sunday morning disturbed and upset, but with a sense that, in her sympathy for the experiences of adolescence, she had found something that might influence her future in nursing.

Meanwhile, February saw the group moving on to consideration of children with learning difficulties and special needs. 'Learning difficulties' means what it says: children whose development is slower than average, or interrupted. The reasons for this might be emotional (children who have been abused often have learning difficulties) or clinical, such as mental handicap. 'Special needs' children may have behavioural problems or a specific disability like deafness, blindness or lack of mobility, which means that they need special help in order to fulfil their potential.

The group now went on more school visits, but this time they were special schools. In the middle of the month, Rachel went to one which particularly impressed her, Oak Manor for blind and visually impaired pupils. 'It was absolutely wonderful. It was near Richmond and the building was gorgeous, everyone was friendly and the children were a smashing bunch. I went with another girl from the group; it was organized through their school nurse – now *her* role is absolutely brilliant. She's based there and she has so much autonomy – she actually has a drugs trolley in her room. She's using her knowledge. She organizes people to come and chat to the children about AIDS, for instance.

'There were eighty-two children, from five to eighteen. We spent a lot of time chatting to the nurse: she showed us her files and what was wrong with the children. The first class we went into had only three girls, who were doing typing. I started chatting to a girl of about twelve. She was using the computer, using the mouse and drawing a picture on it. She wasn't completely blind; I was asking her about it. She was so together about it. She said she could see colours and she could see me, but she couldn't describe me. But she'd know me if she saw me again from my footsteps and my voice – after speaking to me once.

'Both the other girl and I came away with the impression that all the children's other senses compensate for their sight. They touch you and they know you. It made me feel inadequate because I didn't notice those things, and because I take so many things for granted, like making a cup of coffee. One of the boys made me coffee – he asked if I wanted one and I stopped and thought, because I didn't want him to burn himself, but he was perfectly capable of it and it was a lovely cup of coffee.

'They were so much more outgoing than other children, because they have to be. They ask you questions all the time because they have to, they can't see you, whereas other children just look and will recognize you again.'

Oak Manor is a state school. The children board during the week and go home at weekends. They are drawn from a wide area; Rachel met pupils from Buckinghamshire, Berkshire and even West Sussex. The curriculum includes straightforward academic subjects (pupils take GCSEs) and lessons adapted to the children's needs: the children with the least sight, or none at all, are taught to use braille computers. There are also lessons in practical subjects like cookery and in social skills. The aim of the school is to enable the children to lead fulfilling, independent lives. Sadly, this is not always possible. Many of the children at Oak Manor have become blind through serious illnesses like brain tumours. Some of them recover; others don't. While Rachel was with the school nurse, a thirteen-year-old boy came to get his medicine. He had an inoperable brain tumour; after he left the nurse told Rachel that he didn't have long to live.

The morning was spent with the school nurse; during the afternoon, Rachel and her friend were with the mobility teacher. They followed a girl who was going out on her own for the first time, using her cane. The girl had been practising walking alone in the school grounds and she had been out in the streets in the company of staff, but this was the first time that she was to walk alone beyond the school bounds. She was going to a shop to buy two packets of extra strong mints, a trip which involved crossing two main roads. Keeping out of earshot (she didn't know she was being watched), they followed her along the route, ready to intervene. It wasn't necessary. She navigated her way along pavements, across the two roads and into the shop; then the return journey: all done slowly and very carefully, and without mishap.

Afterwards, the mobility teacher asked a couple of boys to show Rachel and her friend round the swimming pool. Swimming at Oak Manor is supervised, but children are encouraged to get themselves in and out of the water alone. On their way round the school, Rachel saw some children being led by others. It could take a long time to find your way around, the boys explained, but ultimately all were working towards independence.

When I spoke to Rachel just after her visit to Oak Manor, she was rhapsodic about it. It was partly relief – she had been worried that she wasn't enjoying her training enough, and kept hoping that coming on the child branch wasn't going to prove a mistake. Now she'd been on a stimulating placement, she felt much better. But it was a shame it had lasted just one day.

By contrast, the start of the year was giving the adult branch students plenty to think about. They had finished their December placements just before Christmas and gone on holiday. The New Year saw them back in college, each embarking on a brand new placement.

Maternity, elderly care, men's health, women's health, and the community were the areas which the students' placements had been designed to cover during the early months of the adult branch. Because of the size of their intake (sixty of them), the students had been divided into smaller groups and were doing the placements in rotation. They had now each completed three of the five placements and had two left to go before April, when they would start rostered service.

They all looked forward to rostered service with a combination of anxiety and excitement: it would mean their being counted as regular members of staff and being given duty rotas on the same basis as everyone else. They would have to do up to ten days on duty at a time – their stamina would be tested, as well as their competence and their ability to become part of the fabric of a ward.

Meanwhile, they had a little over two months in which to add to their knowledge and develop their skills. As before Christmas, their current placements involved ten days on a ward (or in the community), spread over a period of four weeks. This worked out as two or three days on duty each week – the other days being taken up with lectures or independent study. Besides the practical work, students had a fairly heavy programme of study to get through during the next two months, including a written project.

In March they would have two weeks' holiday, in April they would begin rostered service and in May they would sit an important exam. With these milestones now in clear view, the students shared a sense that they were racing to pack in as much experience as they could.

The last placement of the old year had given two of the students, Corinne and Angela, much food for thought: they had both been on the maternity ward in Wavetree District General. This had been an important placement for them, given their plans to go on and train as midwives. How had they got on?

Corinne had enjoyed most of it. She had liked being on the ward and found the midwives friendly. She had taken to working with babies and, like most people, had loved helping at a birth.

Angela had more mixed feelings. She had started the placement on an ante-natal ward, where pregnant women with complications were staying under observation. Most of the complications were fairly minor and therefore not particularly interesting clinically; the most rewarding part of being on that ward was watching the patients, who, Angela felt, were impressively calm under the circumstances. Moving to the post-natal ward and helping to care for newborn babies was more taxing. The mothers were often exhausted from the birth and some were very anxious. At first Angela had felt under-prepared and under-supervised: one day she was left for four hours on her own to supervise six mothers and their newborn babies. 'I was terrified. I had to do general observations, take pulse rates and temperatures. No one had ever shown me how to take a baby's temperature [under the arm] or told me that you measure their pulse rate by heartbeat not by wrist pulse.'

Part of the problem, Angela felt, was that the midwives

on the ward had an ambivalent attitude towards students. 'They're very anxious not to be considered nurses. That means that they can be rather unwelcoming to nursing students.' To be fair, she admitted that this was something of a generalization and, towards the end of her placement, when she went on to the delivery wards she had found the staff more encouraging.

Corinne had no complaints about the midwives she had worked with. And even while Angela criticized the midwives' attitude, she conceded that they had a point: 'I can see why they're miffed to be considered as nurses – they have an extra eighteen months' training; they get a lot more responsibility than, say, a D grade staff nurse. And yet they get graded exactly the same as the regular staff nurse, with no recognition for the difference.'

Lack of professional status notwithstanding, Angela had emerged from her maternity placement still keen to do midwifery. Like Corinne, she had thoroughly enjoyed being present at a birth: 'I cried! It was so wonderful!'

Although they had been on maternity placement at the same time, Angela and Corinne had had little opportunity to compare notes. The shift system and the number of wards within the maternity department had meant that they were never working alongside each other. This was very common among students on placement; most people liked to be on a shift with someone from their set, but it hardly ever happened. Moreover, the students found that it was quite rare even to be on the same placement as people they knew. The seven students in this book had seen quite a bit of each other on the CFP; by the time they were half way through the branch, most of them would be only vaguely aware of where the others were working.

In January, Corinne went on a men's health placement at the Wavetree. Angela was allocated a women's health placement at a private hospital, Heath Hall. Meanwhile, the other students were similarly scattered: it was Emily's turn for maternity, Tim was on an acute elderly care ward at Alf's and Jane was out with a community nurse.

Heath Hall was something of an eye opener for Angela. Being a private hospital, she discovered, meant more than simply having adequate funds for nursing care: it changed the nature of the relationship between nurses and patients.

She was put on a women's ward where most of the patients had come in for hysterectomies. Staffing levels were excellent: each patient had a staff nurse of at least D grade to look after her; named nursing was practised and no nurse was responsible for more than four patients. Angela was told that the number of patients a nurse was given depended on their level of dependency; four surgical patients were considered quite a heavy load, whereas on a medical ward a nurse might be allocated six.

To Angela, used to NHS wards, this was impressive. 'It means that you really can give whole care to each of your patients. In the NHS wards I've been on, you're given about twelve patients. Among them you have those who are supposed to be your special patients, but often you have the auxiliaries give baths, or let someone else do lunches, because you just don't have time.'

It is a long-standing characteristic of the NHS to have a wide skill mix on the wards. Nursing care can then be divided up into tasks and parcelled out, according to the level of skill required. Under this system, sisters or experienced nurses at E or F grade perform, or at least supervise, the more clinically complex tasks. Registered staff nurses (D grade and upwards) are responsible for procedures such as taking observations, changing dressings and administering drugs. Care assistants (people with six weeks' training) or other auxiliaries give baths, help patients dress and serve lunches.

The stated aim of modern nursing is to move away from this approach. Studies show that patients respond better when given all round care by one or two nurses. And all round contact is now recognized as an important aid to nurses when monitoring their patients' condition. Unfortunately, registered nurses with three years' training cost more to employ than care assistants with six weeks', and NHS hospitals, forced to operate within their budgets, are increasingly going for the cheaper option.

Even as Project 2000 trains new nurses to give skilled, holistic care, it becomes harder for NHS hospitals to afford it. Angela felt that in Heath Hall she was for the first time seeing the principles of Project 2000 in action.

Because staffing levels were good, there was little stress among the nurses and they were friendly to her. There was plenty of time for her to ask questions and learn things. The hierarchy she found so irksome in the NHS was hardly in evidence; instead she found a refreshing open-mindedness on the subject of backgrounds and qualifications.

'The staff were great – they were all for foreigners! There were so many Australians and Americans and New Zealanders. And other people who, interestingly enough, had been shunned by the NHS for one reason or another. There was one woman who had trained in the army. She'd been a nurse for twenty years, practising in Germany. She'd come back to this country two years ago and they'd said, 'Well, we'd have to start you at D grade [equivalent to a newly registered nurse]. And we don't want you anyway because you trained in the army and deserted the NHS.' And then this other woman, who was Welsh, had gone to Australia. She had an orthopaedics speciality, and then she'd gone on into a paediatrics speciality – she had really gone up quite high. Again, when she came back the NHS wouldn't recognize any of it. The NHS is *so* peculiar!

'Then there were people on permanent nights, to allow them to be at home during the day. You can't do that on the NHS. They can be so inflexible, it's really sad. A lot of these people didn't want to be working in private medicine, but there's just such a bias against them in the NHS.'

She found that relationships between staff and patients were different in the private sector too. 'The patients at Heath Hall are consumers and they see themselves as consumers, so they're very demanding. It's good, because they ask a lot of questions and you feel you're giving them all the information they should be having and they're actually making autonomous choices. Whereas on the NHS you feel that sometimes people are being coerced because there's just not the time to give them the choices. And they're *so* grateful in the NHS.

'In a way I found it difficult at first at Heath Hall, because you don't have that power thing you're used to in the NHS. Patients are more your equals, and you have to build a relationship with them on a different footing. It's more challenging.'

Angela was able to get to know the patients. She spent a lot of time with one in particular, Caroline, a woman with fibroids in her womb who had come in for a hysterectomy. Angela talked to her before surgery, when Caroline seemed quite happy and settled about the operation. She attended the operation itself, which took much longer than expected owing to the size of the fibroids and was performed with instruments which shocked her: 'It was brutal! They looked like something from medieval times. Honestly, there was this huge *corkscrew* thing!' And she was on hand afterwards, when Caroline became very distressed.

'Everyone was saying, "She's been too together about it, she needs to let it come out," and I think that was true. About two days after the procedure she was very depressed and needed a lot of reassurance and talking.' It was satisfying for Angela to have the time to help her. She had learnt the importance of holistic care on her NHS course; it had taken a private hospital, with good resources, to allow her to practise it.

*

BACK AT ALF'S, on Leonard Ward, Tim was discovering the 'make do and mend' version of NHS nursing. Leonard is an acute ward for elderly people: patients come in with a range of conditions associated with old age, strokes, chest infections, heart attacks and falls being some of the most common. The patients' general physical condition tends to be poor: not only old age, but socioeconomic factors like bad housing and malnourishment have often played a part. And patients often suffer a degree of mental confusion, especially if they have had strokes.

The nurses' workload, therefore, is heavy. Leonard is one of St Alphege's old wards: long, high-ceilinged, with women's beds down one side, men's down the other and a partition in between. When Tim was there, all of the eighteen beds were occupied. Patients who were well enough to move were encouraged to get up every day; as all of them were frail and some were severely incapacitated, this in itself was no small operation.

It was soon evident to Tim that Leonard Ward did not have enough staff to cope. From the beginning the students on placement (who comprised not only those from Tim's intake, but also more advanced RGN students and more junior Project 2000 ones) were being unofficially used as auxiliaries. 'Sometimes there'd be only one trained member of staff and up to seven or eight students on a shift. Obviously, that one person couldn't be responsible for all the students, so the students just got on with it. We tended to be put on morning shifts which meant helping patients get out of bed, washed, dressed, shaved. We made their beds – some of them may have been incontinent. By the time we'd done all that, it was usually nearly lunchtime.'

It wasn't much of a learning experience. The students weren't assigned mentors and on many of the busiest shifts Tim just had to watch the most senior RGN students and be guided by them. He hoped that he was picking up good practice, but had no real way of knowing.

More worryingly, trained staff were so thin on the ground, and so hopelessly busy, that they did not have the time to supervise everything the students did. 'The patients would get split into three teams of six. Sometimes I'd be allocated a team to take charge of myself – I'd be looking after six patients with the help of a care assistant. The RGN in overall charge of the ward would be busy with admin: liaising between the medical team and nursing team, talking to physiotherapy and so on. In the end the other students and I were writing up the care plans ourselves, and they weren't being checked.'

The trained staff who were on the ward were good, Tim felt, and very committed. But there were simply too few of them. 'I'm not saying the care's bad. But potentially it could be bad, because there's not enough people there to check what's being done. I don't want someone looking over my shoulder all the time, but I'd like some supervision.'

It was no great surprise to Tim that Leonard was short-staffed. The underfunding of elderly care is so widespread within the NHS that it has become a simple fact of life. And it's not just hospitals: lack of provision begins in the community and gives rise to a chain reaction in which hospital wards are only one link. Poor living conditions, overstretched GP services and a lack of back up in the community mean that elderly people's health deteriorates and they have to be admitted into hospitals. There they are treated for specific ailments, but pressure on hospital beds means that they are often discharged before they are fully fit. They go back to unsatisfactory living conditions, with little support, and become ill again. They have to be readmitted to hospital . . .

Leonard Ward had its share of 'revolving door' patients that winter. One was Kitty, a woman in her seventies who had been admitted on to different wards at Alf's twice in the previous two months. This time she had come into Leonard via Casualty, after having a fall at home. She had been lying on the floor for a couple of days before anyone found her, and was dehydrated and incontinent and had pressure sores. Doctors also diagnosed border-line malnutrition and a urinary tract infection which required antibiotic treatment.

These days, care of the elderly in hospitals is carried out not by doctors and nurses alone, but by a multidisciplinary team which includes occupational therapists, physiotherapists and social workers. The aim of the team is to restore the patient to health and to liaise with community workers to ensure that when the patient returns home, she or he has adequate support. The latter half of this is known as discharge planning. Kitty's discharge had already been planned twice by St Alphege's; clearly she was finding it more difficult to cope at home than the staff anticipated.

While on Leonard, Kitty's care consisted of rest, regular turning and treatment for the pressure sores, extra fluids and nutrition, and antibiotics for the infection. She also had physiotherapy to get her walking again. She recovered well. She had been confused on admission but that was caused by the infection and dehydration; after two weeks on Leonard she was stronger, the infection was gone and she could walk about with a frame.

Meanwhile, the team was addressing itself to her discharge planning. Liaison with social services had established that Kitty lived alone, had visits from a home help three times a week and received Meals on Wheels twice a week. This was considered a fairly good level of provision and the staff knew Wavetree Social Services would be unlikely to increase it. The occupational therapist visited her flat and confirmed that there were no dangers such as loose carpets or problems like inaccessible sinks. Kitty was recommended for discharge.

It seemed clear to Tim that Kitty didn't really want to go

home. Life there was lonely, she'd never been married and had no real friends; her only visitors were the home help and Meals on Wheels. She was a gregarious person and loved chatting to everyone on the ward. Tim had talked to her a good deal during her stay. 'She really wanted company. She'd be happy to sit and talk to you all day. I talked to her when I could but I was usually busy doing tasks around the ward. Occasionally after lunch I could sit and chat to her. She told me she'd been a machinist, a tailoress. She'd made clothes and hats. She was always very pleasant and if anything, over-grateful for anything you did. "Thank you very much, you're so kind." "Did you enjoy your dinner?" "Oh, it was absolutely wonderful!" You'd think she'd eaten cordon bleu. The hospital food's quite good, but not that good. Perhaps she thought if she was really nice to us we'd let her stay.'

When Kitty was told she'd be going home, she made little fuss. But she kept asking who would be at the flat to meet her, so Tim arranged for the home help to be there. The next day she was packed and waiting to go, ready if not enthusiastic. In the end, she had a brief reprieve because the transport department failed to send anyone to pick her up and once it got dark, the nurse in charge of Leonard Ward decided she would have to stay another night.

'She was really quite pleased. She said, "Will I be going home tomorrow?" I said yes. She said, "Oh well, I suppose I have to." I tried to explain that hospitals were for sick people and she wasn't sick any more and they might need the bed for someone who was. She said, "Oh yes, I understand that. Quite right too. I'll go home tomorrow. I'll be fine." But she kept asking who'd be there.'

Once more, Tim arranged for the home help to be at Kitty's flat, and the following day the transport arrived and she duly went home. Four days later, Tim was unamazed to see her on Leonard: she'd fallen again. 'Whether it was a deliberate fall, I don't know. She wasn't stupid and she could have equated falling with getting into hospital, being fed and looked after and having lots of company. And who can blame her?'

What Kitty really needed, the staff concluded, was some kind of sheltered accommodation. 'Her own space,' was the general consensus, given that she was quite independent-minded. 'Her own bedroom and kitchen area and bathroom,' in Tim's words, 'with a common room she can go to and panic buttons and a warden.'

This was the nursing staff's vision of what Kitty needed. But when Tim's placement ended, no one had yet sat down and talked to her about it. This was caused partly by simple lack of time and partly by a reluctance to broach such a sensitive subject with her. She might find the idea abhorrent; many elderly people do. On the other hand, she might embrace it with enthusiasm, only to discover that nowhere could be found for her. Sheltered accommodation of this kind is in very short supply. The theory of care in the community is that elderly people can be looked after by neighbours, friends and relatives with support provided by social services. But when friends and relatives are few, neighbours are unwilling or unable to help and social services are already providing as much as their budgets allow, what happens to people like Kitty?

Tim finished his placement on Leonard with a growing sense of unease about the the direction of the NHS. He was also anxious about his course work. A project on elderly care was compulsory and he had decided to do a care study on a patient currently on Leonard: a woman with pulmonary embolisms, for whom the medical staff were trying various treatments. But he had found it hard to clear any time in which to study her.

'Once the consultant was discussing her care on the ward round and I was listening, and the staff nurse said, "I know you want to listen to the consultant, but can you just go and bath so and so because she's going home soon." I said, "I'm sorry, I'm doing a care study on this lady, it's really important I listen to this." She said, "Yes, but the ambulance could come for this lady at any time." I said, "Yes, I'm sorry too, but I'm a student and I'm here to learn and this is very important. I'll bath that lady as soon as I've finished here." She kept going on: "But what if the ambulance comes?" I said, "Look, I'm here to learn, I'm supposed to be supernumerary. If you're short-staffed, phone the agency."

'And that was it. She never spoke to me again after that. Never ever. But I had to stand up for my rights there, I had to be assertive. I *am* here to learn. It didn't do much good though – I didn't get the chance to talk to the lady again, I was always too busy and I had to abandon the care study.'

Most students, Tim had found, were reluctant to complain or voice misgivings to staff. However, all the students on that placement felt hard done by, and before they left they put their case to the ward manager. They also agreed that they would mention the staffing problems in their written evaluations on that placement, which they would submit to college.

Tim moved on with relief to his next placement: it was his turn, finally, for maternity. He nurtured no great ambition in that area but he had heard good reports about Wavetree maternity and had no fears about the midwives: 'I know some people say they're very unfriendly and hate nurses, but my male colleagues have mostly had good experiences with them. Maybe they're trying to get men to join. There are only fifty-six male midwives in the country, so we've got novelty value.'

CATHERINE FORD became a mental health nurse by chance. It had seemed to offer a way out of conventional nursing, which she disliked; it also gave her an opportunity to use her degree in social psychology. She had been twenty-six when she began the eighteen-month mental health course at Alf's. It had proved a testing time for her – in fact, most of Catherine's twenties so far had been difficult and her experience of nursing turbulent.

Catherine had grown up in Wales and gone to university in the Midlands. An eccentric mix of science and art A levels, rather than any great sense of vocation, guided her towards her social psychology degree. Throughout her time at university, she kept up a close relationship with her childhood sweetheart back at home and they were planning to spend more time together after she graduated. At the end of her course, however, Catherine suddenly felt she was too young to settle down and decided to go to London and train as a nurse 'partly to get away. Also, I thought nursing would give me a good practical qualification, and then I could go off and travel.'

In what she describes as 'an emotional state', Catherine applied to various London hospitals and was accepted at one in the neighbouring district to Alf's. Because she had a degree, her RGN training was slightly shortened to two and a half years rather than three years and three months. However, it still felt far too long for Catherine, who, to her dismay, found it difficult.

To cut a long story short, Catherine had registered and worked as an RGN in a series of jobs, during which she had become increasingly disillusioned and frustrated. In particular, she had done battle with one sister over what she saw as the rigid hierarchy imposed on staff nurses. She had considered leaving nursing altogether but instead had done an extra eighteen months' training to become an RMN (Registered Mental Nurse). During the training a number of things had gone wrong in her personal life, including her father becoming seriously ill; at work, it was suggested that because of the strain she was under it might be prudent to leave the course. She refused. After having to take some months out when her father died, she finished the course, took a job on a mental health ward in a London district hospital, then applied for a job on Wilcox, a brand new acute mental health ward which had just been built at St Alphege's. She got it.

In January, Wilcox Ward was two years old and Catherine had been a staff nurse there since the beginning. Most of the original nursing team were still there with her and working relationships were good. Catherine was particularly fond of the charge nurse, Malcolm. (Charge nurse is the title given to a male sister.)

Although Wilcox has now seen quite a bit of action, it still looks impressive. It is a twenty-bed unit, with a dormitory ward, two-bed bays and a number of activity rooms, day rooms and offices. It occupies the second floor of a wing in Alf's main courtyard. Entering this wing is an experience rather different from that usually encountered in Alf's: as you approach the entrance, automatic doors open to admit you and close behind you. The floor is carpeted, the walls are painted light blue and there is a lot of pine trim around. The ambience is comforting and hushed. The wing also houses oncology wards and the radiotherapy unit.

Wilcox is designed to be welcoming and secure. Behind the automatically closing doors, the unit has the atmosphere of a social work drop-in centre. Nursing staff wear their own clothes and the various rooms (activity, interview, group rooms, etc.) tend to have noticeboards up, with notices to staff and patients and information about the services available in the community.

There are two consultants attached to the unit and between them they attract a wide range of patients. One consultant is linked to the St Alphege's and Wavetree District Health Authority, and patients are referred to him from the community. They tend to be people on low incomes, often living in poor housing and beset with the social problems that accompany it. A good many of them are from Wavetree's sizeable African Caribbean community. Homeless people (who often became homeless in the first place when their residential provision closed down as part of the move towards care in the community) are also referred. These patients tend to be diagnosed as suffering from depression, schizophrenia or psychosis.

The other consultant is a 'liaison psychiatrist', who works in conjunction with the general medical wards and outpatients clinics at the hospital. If patients on the general wards break down, they will be admitted to Wilcox; patients coming in to the outpatients clinics, on referral from their GPs, will sometimes also be ill enough for admission. The consultant also runs a special clinic for sufferers of chronic fatigue syndrome (CFS) or ME, and Wilcox often has one or two of these patients in for intensive treatment. It is often middle-class, sometimes professional, people who attend the clinic for CFS/ME. Meanwhile, the majority of GP referrals are for general mental health problems such as depression, anxiety or psychosis. In addition, people will sometimes be referred with obsessive compulsive disorders (constant handwashing, for instance), or the eating disorders anorexia and bulimia.

Consequently, the ward has patients from a wide range of backgrounds, with a diversity of conditions. While in Wilcox, most of them take some form of medication – NHS treatment of mental illness is heavily reliant on drugs. Much of the rest of their care is in the hands of the nurses, overseen by the doctors, true, but mental nurses have a great deal of autonomy in the care of their patients. On Wilcox the nurses are split into four teams, each looking after a group of patients. Within the teams, there is a named nurse policy, so that each patient has a named nurse who looks after him or her for the length of the stay. This is vital, because the role of the mental nurse on Wilcox is to work continuously with the patients, helping them to identify strategies for coping with – or at least living with – their problems. The daily routine of the ward is deliberately left unstructured, so that nurses can be flexible with their time and attention.

Catherine described her job as being 'a jack of all trades. I might be doing all kinds of things, from helping someone have a bath to holding an informal discussion session. A lot of it is talking to people and letting them talk to you. As a mental health nurse, my role includes "informal counselling", allowing clients to ventilate their feelings. I am also there to act as their advocate, which sometimes means putting their case *against* the wishes of the medical team.'

Inevitably, given that patients live so close together here and staff spend so much time with them, the ward generates its own emotional currents. Part of the nurses' job lies in coping with these. 'When there's some kind of negative atmosphere building, everyone feels it. The patients are twitchy and unhappy, staff are disgruntled. The ward is like a little ecosystem and its therapeutic atmosphere varies. What happens among patients affects staff and vice versa – we all live here.'

In January, however, Catherine was not sure that she wanted to go on living in Wilcox. True, she had enjoyed working there for the last two years. She liked the relatively unstructured approach to work and she felt that she fitted well into this nursing team. But she had an unfocused sense that she should be doing something else; she should be moving on, trying harder . . .

When I met Catherine, she talked about herself in much the same terms as she talked about her patients. She said that she had had 'a rotten twenties' and identified herself as someone who rushed into things; who, when they went wrong, became very stubborn and wouldn't give up; who periodically had crises of confidence and who experienced problems with authority.

On the one hand, she felt that this made her a better

nurse: 'Because I've been unhappy I can empathize with the patients. I do feel that many good, warm mental health nurses have difficult personal histories of their own.' On the other, it made it very difficult for her to settle.

'This is the best place I've worked and I certainly don't regret coming here. But there are a lot of issues about the nurse's role that I'm still trying to resolve for myself. I feel that nurses should be given much more respect as professionals – on the other wards I've worked on, I've often been in trouble with the sisters for speaking out about things. Even here, a while ago, it happened again. There was a teaching session with a consultant; he wasn't making any sense and everyone was confused, but because he was a consultant, no one liked to say anything, they just sat there and let him carry on. I said, "Hang on, Prof. I'm sorry, but you're talking in riddles." Everyone gasped, and afterwards I was hauled up by Malcolm and he told me that I had been inappropriately aggressive and I couldn't talk to the doctor like that.

'I said, "Why not? I'm sure the Prof didn't mind. I'll check with him to see, shall I?" Malcolm said, "Oh no! Don't do that!" But I did. I called him up and introduced myself and said, "I was the one who asked you to explain things again at the teaching session, I hope I didn't offend you." He said, "No, of course not." And I really don't think he did, why should he?'

The obligation to constrain herself and watch what she said irked Catherine. Things had improved recently, with the departure of one member of staff who had particularly disapproved of her assertiveness, but Catherine still felt restless. Just before Christmas, her partner, Bob (also a nurse), heard that there was a vacancy for a nurse in a community-based 'transition team' in the Wavetree borough. The job would involve assessing patients who were coming into the borough from outside, and those already in the borough who were due to leave acute wards and would require either sheltered accommodation or support to help them live at home. Bob thought Catherine should apply for it; so did she.

Her application had gone in over the New Year and Catherine was invited to go for an interview in a couple of weeks' time. Meanwhile, through various channels (including the staff network on Wilcox), she was receiving encouraging feedback. Malcolm had encouraged her to apply; the selection panel liked what they had heard. The word was that she was the favoured candidate. Catherine therefore began the New Year on Wilcox with very mixed feelings. How long would she be staying here and how much did she really want to leave?

There was a typically mixed batch of patients in at the moment. Some had been admitted for the first time; others had very long histories of mental illness and were well known on Wilcox. One of the latter was Wilberforce, a West Indian man in his fifties. He was diagnosed as a paranoid schizophrenic and had been in and out of hospital repeatedly.

'He has fixed, grandiose delusions which are very hard to change. He can become very aggressive. He's come back in now because he argued with the staff at the residential home he'd gone to. He thought he was in charge of the place and he did things like go out and buy a whole lot of shopping for the other residents. Then he wanted to be refunded and when the staff argued with him he became aggressive and threatened them. So they said they wouldn't have him any more and he's come back into hospital.

'When he first arrived back, the multidisciplinary team assessed him and decided his mental state could be improved by a change of medication. All his symptoms got worse! So they've changed him back and now he's his normal, grandiose self again. We can't do much for him: he lives here like a lodger really. I'm his nurse, so I talk to him about what kind of place he'd like to move to, what he needs and then discuss it with the social worker. But mostly I just spend time with him.'

Catherine was named nurse to one other patient too, a woman called Rhona, newly admitted. She was very different from Wilberforce on almost every count. She was in her early thirties, white, a senior registrar at a neighbouring hospital, with no history of mental illness.

'She's always been a coper, Rhona, but when she was thirty she began to feel that life was passing her by. She was depressed that she had no partner, then she was off sick for a while and that started her worrying about her job security. She got very depressed and took an overdose. That's when she was admitted.

'We developed a programme of tasks for her to do every day, and she's been seeing a psychotherapist. A lot of issues around her family and in particular her father have come up. The staff all felt it was important that continued, so she's stayed in for six weeks. I've been building a relationship with her, having sessions when we talk about all sorts of things that come up.

'Rhona won't be here much longer now. We're trying to encourage her to leave as soon as possible, as the longer she stays the harder it'll be for her to get back to her own life. She finds it very comfortable here but in the last five days she's started to change a lot. She looks different and sounds different. And she says she feels more herself. She's on the mend.'

This fairly intensive, in-patient work is very different from the kind of thing Catherine would be doing if she got the community-based post. Catherine was not sure how she would take to working in a 'transition team', but she was attracted by the prospect of more autonomy and it would certainly be a good career move, given that mental health care will be getting more and more community-based in the future.

It was not to be. Perhaps it was her uncertainty about the

move taking over; perhaps it was the strain of going into the interview as the publicly acknowledged favourite. Whatever the reason, when the day came, Catherine was overcome by nerves: 'I dried. I just couldn't answer the questions.'

By the time she left the room, Catherine knew that it was highly unlikely she would get the job. But it was still a shock when the rejection letter came. Her initial reaction was just that, shock, and depression. She felt that she had let herself down: 'It was particularly awful in a way, everyone knowing I was the favourite.'

So much for choosing whether to stay or go: now she would just have to stay on Wilcox.

OVER AT ST WENCESLAS, Nicola was surprised to find herself enjoying her new placement. She had been dreading a return to the run-down elderly and mental hospital, remembering all too well her CFP placement on the acute psychiatric ward there.

(The terms 'mental health' and 'psychiatric' mean the same thing when used to describe wards. There is a move within nursing to stop using medicalized phrases like 'psychiatric', which concentrate on the illness, and to favour the more positive 'mental health'. However, doctors and hospital administrations often continue to use the word 'psychiatric'. During the interviews the nurses tended to alternate between the two names. Where it does not risk confusing the reader, I have followed their lead. Interestingly, Nicola and Catherine often chose words differently according to whether they were discussing patients – whom they were reluctant to label – or the ward itself, when they frequently adopted the more medicalized hospital jargon.)

For this stint at St Wenceslas, Nicola would be spending two weeks on Morris. This was a ward for people over sixty-five with functional mental illness, which is mental illness like depression or obsessive compulsive disorder that grows out of circumstances and emotions, rather than organic mental illness such as dementia.

As soon as she arrived, one of Nicola's fears was laid to rest: where the other ward had been cramped and dingy, Morris was large and quite bright. It was a combination of what had once been two wards. Besides a main ward area with beds in curtained cubicles, there were some three- and four-bedded bays and some single rooms. All the patients got up during the day: some stayed on the ward; others went downstairs to the day room; still others went out of the hospital altogether, to day centres.

The patients on Morris were not expected to stay for long periods. Two months was the usual maximum stay, after which they would move on – ideally back to their homes, otherwise into residential accommodation. They suffered from a variety of mental and emotional problems. From reading their notes, Nicola gathered that many of them had a fairly long history of difficulties, which were now growing more severe as they grew older. Sometimes an event like the death of a spouse would trigger a depression or lead to a worsening of symptoms which left them unable to cope. Then they would be admitted.

Nicola was working shifts for her time on Morris, not night shifts, but a rotation of 'earlies' and 'lates'. There were several other students on the ward: three degree students and three Project 2000 CFP students on 'obspar'. Despite this, the ward, like most in St Wenceslas (indeed, like most in mental health and elderly care) was understaffed. Nicola had the impression that morale was quite low.

'The nurses are very varied. Some, I feel, don't have many skills, or else they aren't bothered. They're just there to get away with doing as little as possible. Some have good ideas and keep up with current thinking. But what I don't like at all is that some nurses have a very authoritarian attitude and speak to the patients as if they were children.'

With these nurses, Nicola felt, the old idea of custodial care held sway: 'You're the boss, they're the patient, they do what you tell them.' It wasn't new to her; she had seen it in action before, on general wards, but it occurred to her that perhaps it was especially easy to get away with that approach on elderly wards. 'The elderly do have a more deferential attitude towards people in uniform and people they perceive to be in authority over them. They accept treatment that I don't think our generation will stand for when we reach their age.'

One bright spot was the ward manager, who had been assigned to Nicola as her supervisor. Now in her forties, she had come into psychiatric nursing from general nursing and midwifery eight years before and had risen fast. She realized that changes were needed on the ward, and was tough in the way she went about getting them: every so often she could be seen in her office, ranting at one of the staff. Nicola had her doubts about the effectiveness of this form of management and felt rather intimidated by the woman, but in fact she treated the students well, seeing them as the new generation and telling the psychiatrists that they should listen to the students when they did their ward rounds. 'She pointed out that we had more time to talk to the patients than anyone else did and that we came in with fresh ideas.'

It was a nice atmosphere to work in. Nicola carried out basic nursing care, attended some of the therapy groups run by the occupational therapist and took part in the weekly ward rounds where all the staff connected with a particular patient would meet, discuss the options and invite the patient in to take part in the discussion too. These ward rounds gave her a chance to see the multidisciplinary team in action, for the staff members involved would include not just nurses and psychiatrists, but social workers, occupational therapists and any other professional involved in the patient's care.

She also spent a good deal of time talking to the patients and became particularly close to two of them.

Mrs Green was a Jewish woman who had developed obsessive handwashing rituals. She would wash her hands over and over again, for up to twenty minutes at a time. She had run up such huge water bills in her flat that the water board was sending people round to see if there was a leak. The washing was connected with her religion, she told Nicola: it was very important for devout Jews to keep clean. Yet she was giving so much time to the handwashing that other aspects of hygiene went by the board. Her flat grew very dirty and infested by insects. Her neighbours complained to the management of the block, and they, after a series of fruitless confrontations with her, asked the St Wenceslas registrar to go and assess her. They reported her as obsessive, difficult and incontinent; the registrar's assessment was that she did indeed need treatment. Mrs Green, however, disagreed. Eventually and reluctantly, the registrar sectioned her.

(Sectioning is the correct term for what most people think of as 'certifying' a patient. It derives from various sections of the Mental Health Act, which lay out the procedures by which people can be admitted to hospital and kept there against their will. A section applies only for a limited time, after which it can be renewed if the doctors and a social worker think it necessary.)

Mrs Green came on to Morris as an unwilling patient. She was furious with the medical staff and even more furious a few days later when she discovered that her landlords had taken advantage of her absence to evict her. 'The staff nurses were furious because they could see her staying in the ward for months, simply because she had nowhere else to go.'

Mrs Green wasn't an easygoing person. She thought of herself as much more intelligent than the other patients and wouldn't mix with them. She was demanding with the nurses. Nicola, however, found her fascinating to talk to and the two of them struck up a friendship.

'She tells me about her life in the past, and her job, which had been very important to her. She's a very intelligent lady. She worked as a legal accounts clerk and I think she could easily have been a lawyer but her husband thought it would be too much for her because she put everything into the job. She'd take time off for the Sabbath but would then make it up during her official holidays. Her account of it is that he thought it would be too much for her to study as well. She's very, very impressed by educational achievements and when she's talking about her job she'll mention 'the Old Etonian' or 'the person from Rugby school.'

Nicola didn't mention that she'd been to university in case Mrs Green latched on to the fact and made her a focus for obsession. But she did tell her that she had done A levels and studied languages. 'She talks to me for hours on end about the Old Testament and the laws, teaching me the Hebrew words for things, and about the Sabbath. I enjoy it. She says, "Oh, you have *very* intelligent eyes!" '

Nicola grew fond of Mrs Green, but she could see why the other nurses were not. 'She has very bad leg ulcers and there's one particular nurse who works in the community, Sister Davis, who she wants to dress them. The other day, Sister Davis couldn't come in; instead a hospital-based nurse came to do it. Apparently she didn't do it right and the following night she screamed and screamed. I don't dispute that she was in pain but she screamed and screamed and *screamed* for painkillers. The nurses were getting them for her as quickly as they could, but the screaming! And the poor woman in the bed next to her was really upset. It makes me sad because she has so much to offer really.

'But she is very obsessional in the way she talks. She repeats things over and over again if they've been important to her and she's very keen to show she hasn't lost her memory. I think she's really scared of ending up in a ward for people with dementia. She'll want to tell you what she's read and she'll say, "I've only read it once and I can remember all this." She is obviously very scared.'

Nicola wasn't sure that Mrs Green's problems were being addressed on Morris. The hand washing was going on more or less unchecked and the water she used was so hot that her skin was getting red and raw. One day in nurses' handover Nicola asked how long she should allow the washing to go on before stopping it. All the nurses had different answers – there was no consensus and no planned approach for the patient.

'It's been going on for weeks. I'm about to leave now and they're still assessing her, they still haven't got together and come up with an idea for what to do about the handwashing. I feel that something more definite should be done, but it doesn't seem to me as if they've identified what her main problems are.'

The other patient Nicola got to know well was as retiring as Mrs Green was managing. Hilda Verrey was ninety-two but looked younger; she had been living in a nursing home until recently, when she had taken to her bed, complaining of pains in her abdomen and legs. She had stayed in bed for weeks and become very depressed. The nursing home staff were very worried about her – up till then she had been fit and active – so she was admitted to Wavetree Hospital for tests. Nothing was found and Hilda was transferred to St Wenceslas, to be treated for depression.

Hilda wanted to stay in bed all the time and would always ask the nurses to do everything for her. At first, when Nicola saw them refusing, she thought they were being rather cruel. Hilda repeatedly asked to be pushed around the ward in a wheelchair, but instead the nurses gave her a Zimmer frame and insisted that she walk with it. She had terrible trouble, hardly seeming able to stay upright, and Nicola was sceptical when she was told that Hilda could walk quite well when she chose and only wobbled and shook when staff were watching.

'I thought they were being cruel to an old lady but then I realized it *was* true, because I was sitting in the office one day and I saw her walking, when she thought no one was looking, and she walked perfectly well with the frame. But as soon as someone came along she started rattling as if she was falling.'

There was a co-ordinated approach on the ward towards Hilda, to try and make her as mobile and independent as possible and not to allow her to become bedridden. It was an uphill task. 'She would say, "At my age, why don't you help me with my walking and things? Why do you expect me to do everything myself?" There was one thing I said which I think did jolt her a bit. I said, "If we help you and do everything for you, you'll end up in a wheelchair and that would be worse, wouldn't it?" And she went, hmph, and looked a bit thoughtful and for a moment she vaguely seemed to be admitting that would be worse.'

It was only for a moment, however. What Hilda really wanted was to give up and be looked after, and this desire grew stronger when, after three weeks on the ward, she was diagnosed as having MRSA, the 'hospital disease'. MRSA (Methicillin-Resistant Staphylococcus Aureus) is caused by bacteria which commonly live on the skin and is harmless to healthy people; however, on people whose immunities are low it can get into open wounds and make them very difficult to heal. Once it takes hold in a hospital, it can spread rapidly from patient to patient, so sufferers are usually isolated.

'There's no isolation unit in St Wenceslas, so she just went into a separate bedroom. Of course, she was the very worst person to do this to – she took to her bed again and became very depressed.'

The nurses on Wilcox disagreed about whether this course of action was the right one. Concerns about Hilda's mental state conflicted with anxieties about the physical health of the other patients and rifts formed. Then the domestic staff grew alarmed about Hilda's infectious status: rumours went round that MRSA was similar to AIDS and they began refusing to take drinks or food into her room.

Meanwhile, poor Hilda was being treated by being washed in Betadine, an effective but unpleasantly thick, brown antiseptic lotion. 'It was torture for her, as she was quite shy about her body and hated being washed by a nurse anyway. She said, "Oh, I want to die." She said this quite a lot. In the end it's been a bit of a farce because they brought her out of isolation after two days and I don't think her swabs are clear yet. The whole thing has thrown the ward rather upside down.'

Nicola persevered at trying to encourage Hilda to get mobile again, but it was even harder now. It became difficult to get her to talk about anything other than her physical ailments. 'I get the impression with the elderly very often that it's easier for them to talk about physical things. They're not from a generation that talks about emotions: they've been through the war, they're tough. Physical health is very important to them.'

The fear Hilda felt of losing her physical independence made her anticipate it, even perhaps try to accelerate it. By the end of Nicola's four weeks on the ward, the nurses were giving in and starting to push Hilda round in a wheelchair. There is, after all, only so much benign bullying one can inflict on a depressed ninety-two-year-old before it turns into cruelty.

There tends to be a high level of fear among patients on mental health wards: fear of what is happening to them and fear of what the world might impose. On Morris this was allied with the fear of old age and the inevitable failing of the faculties.

Although Morris wasn't supposed to care for dementia patients, some of the people there were very confused and waiting to go on to a continuing care ward (a long-term ward for elderly people who can no longer live on their own). The patients were grouped so that the more confused ones, who needed the most supervision, were together. It was part of the nurses' duties to make sure they didn't wander off at night and put themselves at risk. It was also part of their care to try and reorientate confused patients towards reality.

Nicola was attempting to persuade one of the more confused women to go to a reminiscence group run by the occupational therapist. 'The approach I'm taking with her is validation therapy: you don't keep correcting people and telling them, no, they're in a hospital, no, their mother's dead. You listen and try to pick up on what they're saying. This woman talks about her past, her family and her sisters; she'll talk in the present tense and I'll talk about it in the past, so I think I'm not colluding with her but I am letting her talk about the things that are important to her. But yesterday when I was trying to persuade her to come to this group, she was saying, "Oh I can't. I've got to pick my sisters up. They'll be waiting for me." And I was stumped! I didn't want to say, "No, you're in your eighties and you're in hospital," so I said, "Oh well, I think you'd enjoy it and you've got plenty of time!" But there was no persuading her.'

Nicola had already attended one of these groups, in which objects and photographs are used to help people talk about their lives and to make links between the past and the present. She had also been to a drama group. Both of these were run by the occupational therapist, though one nurse from the ward was usually present too. Nicola thought they were helpful for the patients, but to her eyes they pointed up the generally low level of activities on the ward. For too much of the time, the emotionally distressed patients were left to their own devices. She didn't have to look far to find the reasons: understaffing and lack of resources. She thought back to her pre-Christmas placement at the Grange, where private money bought the patients all the things the people at St Wenceslas needed, congenial surroundings, good facilities and ample nursing time.

'There's just no comparison. In St Wenceslas the ward is quite bright and the nurses have put up pictures, but there are few resources for activities. Morris is on the top floor, the lift is often broken and the elderly people can't manage the stairs. And there's nowhere in Wavetree to go for a walk, no incentive to go outside.'

By the time she left Morris, Nicola was beginning to feel the gulf between what she was taught in the classroom and what happened out there in the NHS. She wasn't alone; when she spoke to the other members of the mental health branch, she found that they were all questioning aspects of the care they had seen. 'You can see it on study days – we have massive debates about medication, people's rights, whether we're making things worse by bringing people into hospital, the stigma of hospitalization. Why is mental health at the bottom of the list for resources? One of my colleagues is having a hard time at the moment, justifying to herself working in the system as she's experienced it. She feels that she could become a part of it, an agent for social control, working for a system which stigmatizes and labels people. I don't feel it that strongly, but it's certainly a danger to be aware of. We want to do the right thing, but it's so easy to get sucked into the system.'

Nicola had always been in favour of care in the commununity: 'Mentally ill people need to be part of society. It's definitely the right direction to be moving in. Labelling and stigmatizing people by leaving them in hospital denies them any chance of a decent future, but moving them out shouldn't be an excuse to save money. People need *more* care, not less, to survive outside hospital.'

She had already seen the effects of inadequate resources on the wards; now she was feeling apprehensive about what she would find in the community. Her next placement was due to be with a Community Psychiatric Nurse (CPN) in the borough of Wavetree, one of London's most deprived areas.

Meanwhile, she was kept extremely busy with college work, extra reading and attempting to have some kind of social life. She spent much of February on academic work. She was researching and writing up a project on community mental health, which involved doing a case study of a patient she had met before Christmas. And now there was a respite from shift work, she had time off at weekends when she could see David, her boyfriend.

THROUGHOUT THE WINTER months, the Save Alf's campaign made dogged progress. This was a critical period for the hospital's future. The government had designated it a 'consultative period' and, with the recommendations of the Tomlinson Report before it, was seeking the views of professional bodies, interest groups and, of course, financial advisers. The London hospitals had been invited to respond to the plans concerning them.

The chief executive and board of St Alphege's had swiftly decided that some change was inevitable. Rather than set their faces against it, they drew up an alternative to Alf's outright closure: a reduction (or 'streamlining' as they put it) of services provided by Alf's to its specialities – cardiology, cancer and AIDS – plus its accident and emergency department. These would continue to be based at the original St Alphege's site; other properties would be sold off. This option, the board argued, would retain Alf's as a centre of excellence while making it economically viable. The campaign produced a document costing this proposal against that of closing the hospital; it also produced its own figures for the cost of keeping the hospital in its present form, which worked out cheaper than the cost of closing the hospital and providing its services elsewhere.

This approach was criticized by some at Alf's. Many of those who worked on the general side – and some from the specialist areas – felt that the hospital should be fighting to keep itself intact, not suggesting how it could be cut. But criticism was muted. Morale was low, there was a sense of confusion and most of the nurses I spoke to, from ward managers to students, felt that the only course open to them was to get on with their jobs and hope for the best.

For many, getting on with their jobs meant straining to meet efficiency targets. Alf's directors were urging everyone to try and impress the government. Budgetary constraints had never been more important. The hospital was hoping to treat a greater number of patients in a shorter period of time, which meant heavy schedules of day surgery and, on the medical side, an increasing pressure on beds. Many nurses felt that discharge planning was growing too aggressive and that patients were being sent home too soon. In Casualty, a row was brewing about the requirement to assess all patients within five minutes.

Outwardly, however, Alf's presented a united front. The alternative proposal was submitted, along with a strong argument for retaining Alf's in its entirety. A minister from the Department of Health visited Alf's and listened to the board's views. He then came back for a second visit. It was seen as a positive sign that he returned for more, but no one really knew which way the government was leaning.

Meanwhile, the campaign continued. Alf's was organizing a huge petition. Already several hundred thousand signatures had been gathered. Statements of support had come from companies in the St Alphege's and Wavetree district, firms in the area had given free legal advice and help with publicity and there was a steady flow of favourable coverage in the local and national press. As far as anyone could tell, public opinion was well and truly on Alf's side.

But at the end of February, the government announced

that it had rejected St Alphege's arguments. The hospital would not be allowed to continue as it was. The government was looking at three options: a drastic slimming down of Alf's (beyond what the directors had envisaged) to a small specialist unit, *without* an accident and emergency department; merger with another London teaching hospital a few miles away; or complete closure.

However, the government had obviously been shaken by the vigour of the campaign for the London hospitals. Not only Alf's but hospitals across the city were protesting against proposals to close, merge and cut their services. Press comment had been unfavourable to the government: while most people recognized that changes were needed in London's health care provision, the government was seen to be acting clumsily.

The government responded by saying that all decisions were to be put on hold. Nothing would happen to London hospitals until October. Meanwhile, it was commissioning a series of 'specialism' reviews, each to be conducted by a team of experts who would look into the provision of a particular type of specialist care across the whole of London. There would be a cardiology review, a cancer review, a renal review and so on. They would report their findings in the summer and hospitals were invited to co-operate with them.

Once again, it was consultation time. Once again, Alf's future was left in the balance. It was at this stage that, thanks to the instincts of the press, the focus of the Save Alf's campaign turned to Accident & Emergency.

'Accident & Emergency' (A & E) is the official hospital term for what most people think of as 'Casualty'. In fact it is the department which, in most hospitals, comprises casualty and related special treatment rooms like resuscitation rooms. It may or may not be linked with a special emergency admissions ward.

The clinical nurse manager of A & E at St Alphege's,

Sister Janet Moore, had been at the hospital for eight years. At thirty-four, she was young to have such a senior position, but she had spent all her career post-registration in A & E and had been promoted fast. 'I was made up to a sister at twenty-two and a half, after only eighteen months on the ward. That would never happen now,' she states matter-of-factly. 'These days we'd want much more experience. And courses are obligatory now.'

Ironically, although Janet's rise would have taken much longer in today's climate, in many ways she appears to exemplify what the new nurse is all about: she is motivated and keen on education for staff and patients, and takes it for granted that on her ward she is the equal of the doctors.

Janet also has the modern nurse's sense of being on a career path. Slightly bored after three years in her first sister's job, she decided to widen her options by leaving and taking a specialist A & E course. It lasted one year and gave her expertise in trauma, burns and minor and major injuries. When she left she had new practical skills such as plastering and she had learnt how to teach care as well as give it. From that course, she joined Alf's as an A & E sister.

'Having trained in a non-teaching hospital, I thought it would be great to come here. Teaching hospitals have an aura, a personality all their own . . . I found it an incredibly friendly place. I was given credit for the work I'd done and the experience I'd had, and within sixteen months of my coming, the senior sister retired and I applied and was successful in getting her post.'

Since then, both nursing grades and Alf's have been restructured. When Janet joined, the A & E department was part of a large unit which included orthopaedic and trauma wards. When I met her, A & E had gained a higher profile: 'We are now a stand-alone directorate which encompasses this A & E department, the Wavetree A & E department and Rupert French acute admissions ward here at Alf's.'

Janet's official title was now 'Clinical Nurse Manager' and she was the senior nurse in charge of the day-to-day running of the department.

'I think this is the most interesting area you could work in. I've been in it for thirteen years and I've never wanted to change because it changes for you, daily. I don't like the kind of unchanging routine where the patients stay the same and I feel I'm not achieving anything. I like a much faster pace of doing things and being able to use all my skills.

'That's not to denigrate what the girls do on the wards. They work incredibly hard and they are the experts in their field. But here I have to know my psychiatry, my gynaecology, my paediatrics, my trauma, my resuscitation – cardiac arrest doesn't hold any fear for me at all because I have to deal with it all the time. Work here is very unpredictable, you don't know what's going to happen next. There could be a bomb in one of the big stations in half an hour and then you'd see the ward take on a completely different character.

'It's a challenge. It's stimulating and it keeps you up to date with every area that you've learnt in training, or that you've experienced. Including social and religious aspects of looking after patients – we get quite an ethnic mix in here.'

Being a nurse in A & E means being ready to deal with whatever presents itself, whether it's a patient with schizophrenia begging to be admitted or a child badly injured in a car crash; an eighty-year-old with a heart attack or a young woman with a suspected miscarriage. When patients are brought in by ambulance, the ambulance crew will call Casualty en route and tell them what to expect. A nurse will be waiting to assess the patient as soon as the ambulance arrives; depending on the urgency of the case, a doctor from the relevant speciality may also be alerted and ready in Casualty.

When patients bring themselves and report to the reception desk, a nurse comes to see them in the waiting area and assesses their condition. She assigns them an order of priority under a system known as 'triage': priority one means to be seen by a doctor immediately; priority two means to be seen by a doctor as soon as possible; priority three means the patient can safely wait for a doctor, without their condition deteriorating (though their temper might).

What this means is that nurses do a good deal of on-the-spot unofficial diagnosis. They then alert the relevant doctors and brief them on the patients. In the treatment areas, they carry out whatever nursing care of patients is required, including specialist A & E techniques such as plastering.

A & E is a prestigious area of nursing I was told by several non-A & E nurses, sometimes with a touch of resentment. It is high-pressure work, perceived as glamorous by the profession and the public alike. Janet rolled her eyes when I mentioned this and told me a story about a keen young student whose first day's work on the ward had included clearing up after an attempted suicide's stomach pumping: 'A bucket of vomit in each hand. I said, "Welcome to A & E!" '

But she acknowledged that A & E nurses were 'a bit of a breed apart. We do challenge more; we have a particularly equal relationship with the doctors. We're an assertive bunch of people and in many cases we've got more experience than we know what to do with. The junior doctors will come to experienced nurses for advice. And we have one consultant who deals with A & E who's very loyal to us, he'll sway into the frame for us. And I'm very loyal to him. It's a mutual department we're running here. We respect each other for what we know and if we're annoyed at each other we yell. Well, we have "free and frank exchange".'

Janet has a free and frank manner anyway. She is rather less than average height, rather more than average weight and has what male novelists used to call 'fine eyes'. In our first two meetings, my impression was of an entirely professional person, so professional that I could get no feel for her life outside work, despite her telling me that she lived in north

London, mixed socially mainly with a group of people she had known from training and had an amateur interest in archaeology. But on the third occasion she was wearing her own clothes (skirt and jumper) instead of uniform and her hair was no longer pulled back in a bun but had been cut into a loose bob. She looked much younger and slightly mischievous; I think she knew I hadn't recognized her.

(I often found it a shock to see how uniform changes nurses. The students look younger on the wards, because the uniform strips them of their chosen personal style and awareness of their student status takes away their self-possession. The qualified nurses look older at work, as if they put on authority with their hospital clothes.)

To get back to the free and frank exchanges: about ten minutes after Janet had used the phrase, the waves from one such incident burst into her office. There was a knock on the door and one of the A & E junior sisters erupted into the small space, shaking and almost incoherent with rage, and started talking at once; a few seconds later she was joined by another nurse who acted as prompt and chorus.

Apparently, the two of them had been having lunch in the canteen when news came via their bleeps that a patient had fallen off a balcony from one of the wards. The canteen was near the ward in question so they rushed straight there, saw that the man was badly injured and took him straight to Intensive Care, where they called an orthopaedic surgeon. The patient was diagnosed as having a fractured pelvis, a life-threatening injury which required immediate surgery to stop the bleeding. Meanwhile, the orthopaedic surgeon asked for the patient to be put in MAST trousers (Medical Anti-Shock Trousers), which inflate around the legs and divert the blood supply to the vital organs.

The nurses told him that A & E didn't have any. There is controversy about MAST trousers and Janet and her colleagues believe that where surgery is available, use of the trousers can do more harm than good. The surgeon disagreed. He refused to believe the hospital didn't have any. He insisted that the nurses should find them. A violent row ensued. Ultimately the surgeon insisted that a call be put out to nearby hospitals to have some MAST trousers urgently sent over and the nurses had come charging back to A & E to claim Janet's support. She listened to the torrent of words, frowned, nodded, frowned and said she would speak to the surgeon about it.

She seemed unmoved, but when the nurses left and I asked for her opinion on the row, her voice was quite clipped with anger. 'The nurses here are all very well trained. Lots of them – and lots of our doctors – have been through a very thorough course of training in how to treat trauma. We started doing that in the late eighties because trauma is the largest cause of death in under-thirty-fives in this country, and the Royal College of Surgeons brought out a report saying that 2,500 young people were dying unnecessarily of trauma, in hospital, because of inadequate care. So we set out to train people up very, very highly. I can look after a trauma victim. I don't have any trouble looking after them, we do it to an agreed protocol. And for a fractured pelvis, with lots of bleeding, where the patient is already in hospital, MAST trousers won't do any good. I think they're useful *only* when you can't get patients to hospital quickly. Perhaps. This surgeon's got the man in theatre; he needs to put a fixation on the pelvis, see what's causing the bleeding and stop it. Otherwise the man will die. This is an orthopaedic surgeon, I shouldn't have to tell him that.'

In fact, she would have no opportunity to tell him that in regard to this patient; as he was already in theatre, he was out of Janet's jurisdiction.

Senior sisters (or ward managers as they are sometimes called) hold the ultimate responsibility for nursing care in their ward. In Janet's case, this means A & E, including resuscitation rooms and Rupert French, the emergency admissions ward. 'I'm much more on the management side now than I used to be. My responsibility encompasses things from education to nursing policy to clinical matters [e.g. the use of MAST trousers]. I have a counterpart at the Wavetree and we liaise together so that we have a uniform approach to things. I'd say about 30 per cent of my time is now clinical; 70 per cent is spent on management issues such as staffing, on lots of teaching at the college and on site cover.'

Site cover is one of those fascinating aspects of hospital life which insiders take for granted and at which outsiders boggle. Out of office hours, when the administration staff have gone home, responsibility for all nursing and practical matters in the hospital comes to rest on one individual designated as being 'on site cover'. Senior nursing staff take it in turns to do site cover, following the shift system. At St Alphege's, Janet is one of them.

'I quite often do it at the weekend. Basically, you're being senior nurse for the hospital and administrator as well. When I'm doing site cover I can't allow for doing anything else, because it's me, no one else but me, and any queries of any sort are going to come on to my bleep, from the whole hospital. It's quite a change in emphasis and though I've got many years' experience, some of the things they ask me are nowhere near my speciality and I have to say, "I don't know but I'll find out for you." There are very few sisters on at weekends – most wards only have one or two sisters and with the nature of rotation, leave and nights, you can't have a sister on all the time. So the nursing staff and medical staff, when they need support, call the person on site cover. If there was a flood, or a fire, or the lavs were leaking, I'd have to deal with it. And requests for agency nurses, drug errors, going to sort out patients who are complaining, to find out what the problem is. We try to avert a formal complaint but if they have a justifiable complaint, we advise them on what course to take.

'You might get thirty or forty calls on a shift. It depends

on what's going on. Being such an old building, if it rains then everything starts to leak. And if a big event happens, like recently when we had a famous footballer brought in injured, then everything goes mad. The press are relentless in their pursuit of knowledge and our press office is closed at weekends, so all enquiries would come to me. Statements are issued but the press are incredibly devious. They'll put on fake bandages and come in to the treatment area to get a story.'

Janet's attitude to such press antics was one of exasperated tolerance. There had been a media presence in Alf's for several weeks while the footballer was a patient; she had found it quite diverting: 'I remember walking across to the Intensive Care block he was in, for something quite different, and about twelve journalists rushed out at me and said, "Are you going up to see him?" "What's his condition?" "I saw the lights go on in the theatre. Have they taken him back in for more surgery?" I said, "Please, there are four wards in there all sending people for surgery; it could be someone going in to have their squint repaired." I think every Afro-Caribbean looking person who exited the stairs was accosted on suspicion of being a member of his family.'

That had been at the end of last year. This year, so far, the press interest in Alf's had concentrated on its threatened closure. And Janet had not done site cover for months: A & E had been seriously understaffed and she had had to go back on the rota full time, making herself available for clinical work on every shift. She still had to squeeze in her management and teaching activities, cancelling leave and working unsocial hours to do so. The only give in the system was site cover, which she could beg off; and beg off she had done.

The staff shortages had initially arisen because of natural movements – one sister left, another went on maternity leave – but they were then exacerbated by the uncertainty about Alf's future, as the hospital managers, feeling jittery, instituted a near-total job freeze. It took Janet eight weeks to get clearance to advertise the sister's post and when the applications began to come in there were fewer than expected: nurses were wary of coming to a hospital under threat.

However, a replacement sister had now been hired and Janet was able to ease up on her clinical work and give her attention to some pressing management and policy issues. She was also able to look at the figures for patients treated in Casualty during these winter months: they made interesting reading and confirmed a trend she had observed for herself on her shifts.

St Alphege's A & E department treats an unusual mix of patients. About 70 per cent of them are commuters, drawn from the huge population (approximately 3 million) who travel daily into work in this part of London. Most of them work in offices, though there are warehouses and catering businesses in the area too; the latter contribute their fair share of cuts and burns patients, whilst other workplace accidents include falling downstairs and getting caught in machinery. Road traffic accidents (RTAs) account for a steady flow of patients.

Commuters also present themselves in Casualty with a range of minor complaints which could and should have been taken to their GPs. They often come in after weekends with sporting injuries; they even bring their holiday mishaps in once they've returned home. It's an abuse of the casualty service, but the staff know it is almost impossible to eradicate it. They try to discourage these patients: they tell them that they are low priority in the queue to see the doctor, that they will probably have to wait several hours while more urgent cases are seen and that they should make an appointment with their own GPs. It has little effect; people seem content to sit in Casualty and wait – all afternoon if necessary.

The other 30 per cent of patients live locally. The area

just to the north of Alf's is residential, mostly working class, with a high percentage of council housing. Residents come in after domestic accidents and RTAs. Elderly residents in particular often come in to Casualty, not only after accidents but with breathing difficulties and undiagnosed pains. The department sees a number of children too, especially during the school holidays when they are at large and at play.

With local patients too, there is a problem separating the A & E department's role from that of the GP. But in Janet's view this is more often the fault of the GPs than the patients. 'There are a lot of GPs who aren't willing to give the support they should. This part of London has quite a low performance rate from GPs. Some surgeries are excellent but there are others which refer patients here without making any attempt to sort them out. For instance, they'll send them along for X-rays to appease them. Now GPs can organize X-rays themselves and get the reports back – everything's orientated towards sorting the patient out within the community nowadays, but some people are very reluctant to do that.

'The worst thing is that they often send those patients who are most in need of social services' attention, elderly people, for instance. Sometimes we'll talk to the families and find that they've been trying for ages to gee up social services, perhaps to get the person into sheltered housing, and then something happens to bring about a rapid deterioration – a fall or a minor stroke – and the GPs will send them to Casualty.

'Often we'll have to admit them because we'll discover an underlying medical problem which hasn't been addressed by the GPs.'

During recent months, Janet had been noticing some changes in the normal seasonal pattern of A & E patients. The overall number of patients coming in was about the same as in previous winters, but the conditions they were presenting were slightly different. 'Normally this time of year we're full of knee and thumb injuries from skiing. There haven't been so many this year, I suppose people can't afford to go. We've not been very cold this winter so we've not had so many hypothermics in. And people are better educated now about keeping their heating on – I've noticed that changing year by year. It's not been icy so we've not had so many fractured hips, which are usually the most common thing this time of year.

'But it has been damp and we've had *lots* of chest infections. Lots of pneumonias, lots of exacerbations of things like chronic bronchitis, emphysemas. A lot of patients are referred by doctors; others call the ambulance because their condition has suddenly got worse. Most of them need admission and treatment.

'And just recently we've had a huge increase in people with stomach bleeds. This isn't a seasonal thing but has been happening noticeably over the past six to eight months. It's nearly all alcohol-related and I think it's due to the recession having been with us for a couple of years now. People have been drinking and smoking more and the long-term effects of it are now being seen.'

The steady year-on-year rise of two other kinds of patients also continued: people who were HIV positive and the homeless.

These trends had one overwhelming implication for Alf's A & E department: they all produced more patients who needed admission to wards. Finding beds on wards is always a problem for A & E departments and has become much worse since the drive towards cost efficiency began. By definition, the more 'efficient' a hospital becomes, the fewer free beds there are, yet a busy A & E department requires a certain margin in available bedspace, or it can't give patients the care they need. Janet was used to finding her way round the bed shortage at Alf's; since Christmas, however, the high rate of A & E patients needing admission and the squeeze on staff costs meant that the shortage had turned into a crisis.

Patients were regularly spending whole days and nights in Casualty. One night in late February Janet and her colleagues had to care for nine of them: all emergency admissions, sick, weary and distressed, trying to sleep on trolleys while they waited for beds to come free. A few days later, the A & E department learnt that it, together with the chock-full wards, was surplus to London's requirements.

When I spoke to Janet the following week, her reaction to the news was unalarmed. This was partly due to a certain battle-weariness: there had already been so many predictions of radical change, none of which had come to anything; why should this one be any different? But more than that, whatever the government might be planning, the task of running Alf's A & E department day by day continued to be as real, absorbing and immediate as always. It was difficult for anyone working in the thick of it to believe that all this activity might soon cease. I discovered this myself when, early in March, I spent an afternoon there.

The outer lobby of A & E is a busy place, reminiscent of an old-fashioned station. One long, high oblong concourse is carved up into seating blocks, 'refreshment' areas, kiosks selling snacks and various reception and information desks. Doors along the walls have signs above them, indicating different clinics, X-ray rooms and offices. Come in through the swing doors, turn left past the first snack kiosk and you reach a maze of plastic bench seats and stacking chairs, with a reception desk alongside. This is the Casualty waiting area.

In the early afternoon of 10 March it was full. A laminated board gave the names of the consultant and the sister (Janet Moore) on duty and the current waiting times – Priority One: immediate; Priority Two: twenty minutes; Priority Three: one to two hours.

Past the noticeboard an unobtrusive door leads into the Casualty department itself. The layout is hard to grasp at first: there is a square space, with five curtained cubicles around the edges and on the far side the nurses' station (a large counter-style desk with many telephones on the working area and a little office behind). Beyond this is a corridor, with cubicles number six to sixteen on either side and a few more makeshift offices, including Janet's cubby-hole. A broad passage leads away to wards, theatres and resuscitation rooms out of sight.

That day, the department was frantic. The big white board in the nurses' station, divided into squares representing the different cubicles, was thick with notes. Fourteen of the sixteen cubicles were occupied, some by patients waiting to see doctors, others by patients who had been seen, diagnosed and given interim treatment and who were now waiting for beds to come free on wards.

The nurses' station was buzzing. There seemed to be an inordinate number of nurses in the dark blue sister's uniform. Janet, emerging from her cubby-hole and rushing off to a meeting in a different department, paused to explain that because it was so busy, they had pulled in extra nurses who would normally be off duty. She herself was one. She had come in as an agency nurse to make up the numbers. This meant that she was actually being employed at a lower grade and a lower rate of pay than her real one, but she would rather do that, she said, than stay at home as she was entitled to do and hire a stranger at the correct grade, who could not possibly get the same amount of work done. Her unorthodox presence, and that of another sister, meant that there were four sisters on duty instead of the usual two, together with a couple of staff nurses and several RGN student nurses.

There were also many doctors in the department. During my first ten minutes there, I counted five clustering round the nurses' station, being briefed on the patients they had come to see, conferring with nurses about their condition, discussing how best to find them beds and updating the information next to the patients' names on the board.

One doctor, a man in his thirties, confirmed to one of the sisters (Helen, a thin fair woman who looked tired) that he had discharged Mr Hansford. Helen turned to a student nurse and asked her to 'take his line out'.*

Lines have to be put in by doctors, but nurses can remove them; the student nurse went off to do so.

As the doctors arrived and departed and the nurses went on the telephones in relays, trying to find beds, I began making notes on the patients. I had to glean my information from reading the board and listening to the nurses and doctors talking; there was no question of their having the time to brief me. After a while I felt as if my head was on a swivel: there were so many doctors coming and going, nurses conferring with them and each other, and student nurses doing errands round the cubicles, that it was hard to keep track. Whenever a nurse came off a telephone, it would ring within seconds. Communication was fast-paced and relentless and to the outsider looked chaotic, rather like a commodities trading floor.

After a while, I had managed to make these incomplete notes:

CUBICLE 1 – Man, age 45, from Leatherhead. Chest pain – suspected cardiac. Being admitted.
CUBICLE 2 – Man, age 40. Facial injury.
CUBICLE 3 – Elderly woman, had suffered fall. Was here alone. When asked if under stress, said 'no more than usual'.

* A 'line' is a tube which feeds into a patient's vein via a 'cannula', a hollow needle with a plastic surround. The line can be used to give patients intravenous drips or medication.

CUBICLE 4 – Woman, age 70, brought in after fainting. Friend (male) was with her. Doctor had ordered an ECG to be done.

CUBICLE 5 – Empty.

CUBICLE 6 – Empty.

CUBICLE 7 – 3-year-old girl with abdominal pain. With mother.

CUBICLE 8 – Mr Hansford. About to go home.

CUBICLE 9 – Woman who had collapsed while crossing the road and injured her head on the kerb.

CUBICLE 10 – Woman, age 85, who had come in the previous night. To be admitted; awaiting hospital transport to take her to bed in Wavetree.

CUBICLE 11 – P. Ellis, a young woman having a miscarriage. Gynaecologist had ordered a D & C; she was waiting to go to day surgery. She was very upset; her mother was on the way.

CUBICLE 12 – Man who had been here since yesterday.

CUBICLE 13 – Woman. I couldn't find out more.

CUBICLE 14 – Man, late middle age, to be admitted.

CUBICLE 15 – Man, here since last night, to be admitted. A bed had now been found for him, but first a doctor had to come and confirm that he needed admission.

CUBICLE 16 – Man with bad internal pain. A doctor was currently with him; he emerged and told nurses he suspected a kidney stone. The man was to be admitted.

By the time I'd made these notes, I knew it would be impossible to track all these patients through the afternoon. I decided to keep an eye on P. Ellis, the young woman miscarrying in cubicle 11, and to follow other events as and when I could. I soon discovered I was not the only person who was confused.

At about 2.15, Alice, the student nurse who had gone to take Mr Hansford's line out came back and told Helen that she had done so. Ten minutes later, the doctor who had made the initial request emerged from somewhere else in the department, stopped a different student nurse and asked her to take Mr Hansford's line out, as it hadn't been done yet and the patient was waiting to leave. He waited while she went into cubicle 8 to perform the task, then watched as she came back to the nurses' station and wiped Mr Hansford's name off the board. At some stage during the next ten minutes, Mr Hansford left.

At 2.20, a female doctor came to the nurses' station and, speaking at large to the group of nurses there, said that the day ward wanted P. Ellis, the patient in number 11, to go down. I wasn't able to see which nurse exactly acknowledged the message, but someone must have done, as the doctor quickly went away again. I wasn't sure what the message meant, so I began to watch for signs of activity from cubicle 11, but all that happened in the next few minutes was that P. Ellis's mother appeared and asked a nurse something.

At 2.30, a student nurse I hadn't seen before asked Helen if the man in cubicle 1 was staying in, and should she keep up observations? Helen said yes. At this, Alice, the first student nurse I'd noticed, chipped in and said no, surely number 1 was going home; she had already taken his line out. No, said Helen; you were asked to take out Mr Hansford's line, in cubicle 8. Alice went scarlet and covered her face – she had taken out the wrong patient's line. Helen was very nice to her and told her not to worry, when it was as busy as this, instructions got misheard. She sought out the doctor who had just conveyed the message about the miscarrying in number 11, and put her in the picture about number 1. The doctor said 'Get another line put in number 1 a bit later. We don't want to alarm him.' (This was duly done later, but so discreetly that I didn't notice it.)

At 2.50, a very young-looking student nurse with a brown ponytail took P. Ellis's mother to the drinks machine to get some tea. While she was gone, one of the nurses looked at the board and asked if a call had come through for number 11 yet; she was told no. I became slightly bewildered and began to wonder if I had understood that earlier message correctly.

At 3.00, an ambulance brought in a man who might have been anywhere between forty and seventy, and an escort of two young Salvation Army workers. The staff were expecting him as they'd taken a phone call from the Salvation Army workers, saying he was in a state of collapse and they suspected a drug overdose. A young, quick-mannered sister called Debbie tried to find out from them and him what he had taken. He was put into cubicle 6. After five minutes she emerged looking cross: 'On the phone they said he was unconscious with pinpoint pupils and not breathing much. So I told them to call an ambulance and bring him in and he's not nearly as bad as that. He's sitting in a chair, pupils size five, smells heavily of alcohol. And he was in last week too.'

A couple more nurses now began discussing the woman in cubicle 11. She was due to have a D and C (a surgical cleaning out of the womb) in day surgery this afternoon. Had a call come through for her yet? They were told no. I wondered if 'day ward' and 'day surgery' were one and the same.

At 3.15, a male nurse overheard one of these questions and said he'd been at day surgery at 2.30 and the staff there had said they'd be calling A & E to have her sent over. The nurses agreed no call had come, so one of the sisters telephoned day surgery and discovered that it was now too late. Apparently day surgery *had* called through to request the patient be sent to them but she hadn't come and now some members of the surgical team were going home.

By now I had realized that 'day ward' and 'day surgery' were indeed the same. I checked my notes. The doctor who had addressed the group of nurses at 2.20 must have taken the call and had been passing on the message, but the nurses had all been so busy that each had thought the doctor was speaking to someone else and none had heard.

An argument ensued, conducted via phone calls between A & E, day surgery and Gynaecology (a gynaecologist had come down to A & E to examine P. Ellis and had liaised with day surgery) as to whose fault it was. The patient would have to be sent home now and asked to return tomorrow. As she was already very upset, none of the nurses fancied telling her. The sister rang the gynaecologist and said it was her responsibility to tell the patient; the gynaecologist replied that she was too busy to come.

At 3.20 a doctor appeared and said the man in cubicle 1 (whose line was now back in) was to be admitted.

At 3.45, the drunk man in cubicle 6 said he wanted to leave, the Salvation Army workers said they couldn't take him back to the hostel in case he collapsed and Debbie, looking frazzled, had an argument with them for misleading A & E about his condition. They retorted that his pupils had been pinpoint earlier and they couldn't take him home. Debbie said A & E couldn't keep him either. The patient emerged from his cubicle and stumped out of the department, muttering that he was going to have a cigarette. He never returned.

For the rest of the afternoon, in between seeing to other patients, the argument about the woman in cubicle 11 rumbled on. The sister who had made the initial phone call to Gynaecology made many more. She told the other nurses repeatedly that she was determined to get the gynaecologist to take responsibility for this mix up. Meanwhile, the patient stayed in the cubicle, being comforted by her mother and the student nurse with the ponytail.

The student came to the nurses' station several times to

say that the patient – whose name, I now discovered, was Patricia – was very upset and still thought she would be having an operation today. Couldn't someone go and tell her the situation and let her go home with her mother? She asked it tentatively, reluctant to seem to criticize the sisters, but evidently sorry for the patient and unwilling to let it go. Each time she asked, the sister got on the telephone again.

It was easy to see how the misunderstanding had happened, in the mêlée. For the whole afternoon almost every cubicle had been taken and it is impossible fully to convey in writing the ceaseless demands on the nurses' attention. I don't think there were more than thirty seconds at a time when the telephone wasn't ringing. All the same, I shared the student nurse's unease. Accountability is all very well, but what happened to putting the needs of the patient first? Whoever was at fault here, surely the patient should be told the news as soon as possible and be allowed to go home and grieve with her family? I wondered if things would have drifted so far if Janet had been in the department (she was still out at her meeting).

When I finally left the department at five o'clock, Patricia Ellis was still in cubicle 11.

'I THINK YOU will be surprised when you come on to the ward,' Christine Carton said. 'The building is old but inside it's not bad. We try to make a homely atmosphere. The patients have their own dresses, knickers, vests, nightdresses – some of them have their own dressing gown. They have their own toiletries, toilet bag and face cloths. Some of them have their own towels, others use the hospital's. All clothes are marked with their names so they don't get lost in the laundry.'

These everyday details, just as much as clinical matters, are central to Christine's nursing. She works on Hamilton, a continuing care ward for women in St Wenceslas' Hospital. 'Continuing Care' means the care given to elderly people who can no longer look after themselves. They are not acutely ill, although they may have an organic disorder such as Alzheimer's Disease, or Parkinson's, or they may have had debilitating strokes. They may have conditions that need monitoring and medication, such as heart conditions or diabetes. But these are not the prime reason they are on the ward; that is, quite simply, that they are no longer strong enough to look after themselves.

Most people, within the NHS and outside it, believe that these elderly people should not be in hospital. However hard the staff try to make the wards comfortable, a hospital remains an institution and what most people crave at the end of their lives is a home. But there are not enough state-funded residential homes to go round, especially for people who need a high degree of physical care. The people on continuing care wards are not candidates for 'care in the community', even if it were to be properly funded. So they stay in hospitals, while plans to transfer them to new, purpose-built residential units are drawn up, costed and, more often than not, set aside. Ever since Christine came to St Wenceslas twelve years before, there had been talk of the health authority building two new nursing homes in the area, to take at least some of the long-stay elderly patients from the hospital. There had been many false dawns but this spring it did seem that at last something was happening: one of the projects (the one furthest from St Wenceslas) was given funding and building was due to begin.

It would be more than a year before the building was habitable and no indication had yet been given as to where its residents would come from. If Hamilton was to close, then Christine hoped she might be able to transfer with the patients to the new home. Meanwhile, she was seeing in her thirteenth year at St Wenceslas.

Christine is from Dominica. She began her working life as a primary school teacher, then decided to train as a nurse. She chose to come to Britain for the training, because the British qualifications were recognized worldwide and she and her husband were considering travelling. She was married with two small children and it meant leaving them behind with her husband. However, her mother and sisters offered to help care for them, and Christine knew that if she trained in Dominica she would have to work frequent night shifts, which would disrupt the family routine anyway.

She opted for the two-year enrolled nurse course, as it meant a shorter separation. With hindsight, she would choose differently, but at the time no one explained to her the difference between an enrolled and a registered nurse, and she didn't realize that an enrolled nurse cannot progress up the career ladder without undertaking further training and becoming registered. So she came to the UK as one of a group of student nurses in 1969 and returned to Dominica in 1971 as an SEN (State Enrolled Nurse).

There followed a period of working in different disciplines in Dominica: Christine nursed in medical, surgical, gynaecology and paediatric wards. Then her husband went to France to work, and shortly afterwards she followed with the children. She worked in an orthopaedic clinic and then in a general hospital. These jobs gave her valuable extra experience. In Britain at the time, nurses were not allowed to give IV drugs or take X-rays (they still are not, unless they have done the relevant extra training and have the certificate to prove it). In Dominica Christine had already learnt how to give IV drugs and drips; now, at the French clinic, she learnt to do X-rays of the leg.

In the mid-1970s the family moved to Britain and Christine began work at St Wenceslas. In those days, it was not yet part of the St Alphege's group and it had a wider range of patients than now. She worked on a rehabilitation ward for head injuries and strokes, where the patients were mostly under fifty.

Christine is small-boned and rather graceful. She moves efficiently and gives the impression of organizing her time well. If she made slightly more fuss about what she did, she could be called 'brisk', but in fact she gets things done with no bustle at all. She has a quality of stillness which must be restful for her patients, although it is quite disconcerting for someone trying to interview her. The impression of repose is partly the result of concentration: Christine takes her work seriously, whether she is performing it or discussing it.

This has not always been a recipe for getting on well with others. Christine spent five years on the rehabilitation ward, where she liked the work but was not particularly happy with her colleagues. 'I was fed up with the same people all the time,' was how she described it. She was cautious about being drawn further. However, from what she told me later, my guess is that she found some of her colleagues lax and they in turn resented her attempts to raise standards. At any rate, she asked to be moved to care of the elderly, and so came to work on Hamilton Ward.

It is an all-woman ward, with twenty-two beds grouped in bays of four, and there is the usual curtained-cubicle arrangement round each bed. It is a hospital, and unmistakably so, but it appears less institutional than most wards, thanks to the variously patterned quilts and pillows, and the scattering of personal possessions on the bedside cupboards: framed photographs, small vases, an ornament or two. A few beds have small portable televisions next to them.

The ward is spread out around a central corridor: the bed bays occupy two main areas; other small rooms do service as office, cloakroom and staff room; and at one end of the corridor the day room, a large oblong room, opens out. Windows line two sides of the day room, and it gets good natural light. Hamilton is on the fourth floor, giving anyone who cares to look out of the window views of the other St Wenceslas buildings and the roads and council blocks of east London beyond. It is mainly the nurses who glance out as they go about their work.

When I first visited Hamilton, the tables pushed together in the centre of the room bore several vases of forced spring flowers: gladioli, irises and tulips, their edges turning slightly brown but still colourful and cheerful. One by one, the nurses were bringing patients, washed, dressed and breakfasted, into the day room.

The nurses on Hamilton work in teams, with two teams on each shift, dividing the patient care between them. Each team is therefore responsible for the care of eleven patients and within the teams, a named nurse policy operates. Each team has three named nurses and each named nurse has three, four or five special patients, the number depending on their mobility and level of dependency. She is responsible for seeing to all their needs while she is on duty, with help from auxiliaries. This offers continuity to the patients and helps preserve dignity in their dealings with the nurses. It also fosters strong bonds between nurse and patients. The patients on the ward are all called 'elderly' but in fact they span an age range of nearly thirty years: the youngest patient is sixty-seven, the eldest ninety-six.

Christine is a team leader, which means she has eleven patients under her overall care and supervises the work of the other nurses on her team. She also has 'named' patients of her own. In January she had just one out of the three she had been used to nursing: Margaret and Rana had died before Christmas, leaving her with only Lena.

When I first talked to Christine, the loss of those patients was still very immediate. She was, she said, being assigned new people to take on in their stead, Edie and Grace, but she did not know them very well yet. As she talked me through the organization of the ward and the kind of work that constitutes elderly care, she referred back again and again to Rani, Margaret and Lena, describing their personalities and circumstances and explaining the care that they needed. So I've followed her lead: her new patients will figure in later chapters; this one is concerned with the two women she was still mourning at the start of the year, and with the third, whose health was likewise failing.

Margaret, an Irish woman, had been on the ward for two years, having arrived from an acute ward. She was immobile, very obese and doubly incontinent and she couldn't feed herself. She was also very confused and could articulate only her simplest needs. Christine and the other nurses had set about trying to improve her condition. It was a long and painstaking process.

'For the incontinence, we would record the times she had a bowel movement during the day, and we started taking her to the toilet regularly at those times. In three or four weeks we were able to keep her clean – that is, during the day. But at night we couldn't because it's not practical to be taking a patient to the toilet every three or four hours.'

At the same time, they had begun to tackle her obesity. 'It was because of her weight she wasn't walking. We managed to reduce her weight to something reasonable. Then she managed to feed herself, first with a puréed meal, then she went back to a solid diet. She had a nephew who was the only person close to her in this country. He would come to see her and feed her all the time, with cakes and biscuits, so we had to educate him that he mustn't give her anything fatty. Once we had reduced her weight, we made her mobile, with the help of a Zimmer frame and a nurse.'

I was struck by the way Christine talked, with a curious mix of compassion and dispassion. She discussed the mechanics of making Margaret healthier as if they were just that: mechanics. I wondered how Margaret had felt about all this.

'She was so confused, we didn't know how she felt. She

could communicate – she could tell you she wants a cup of tea or a glass of water, but she couldn't tell you how she feels about her mobilizing. She could recognize her nephew when he came and she could recognize the different nurses, though she didn't know them by name.'

In the two years Margaret had lived on Hamilton, she had never been able to put a name to Christine's face. However, Christine knew her patient recognized her and liked her. She had become fond of Margaret too. With the extent of Margaret's confusion, there was little they could have by way of conversation but there are other forms of communication, such as touch, facial expressions and the fact that Christine was the one who day after day worked with Margaret, helping her to look after herself.

When Christine had first come into care of the elderly, thirteen years ago, it would not have been possible to give such consistent care to one patient. In those days, nursing of the elderly was far more task-oriented, with procedures like washing and feeding of patients divided out amongst different nurses. 'I won't say the elderly people were ill-treated, but they were seen like a piece of furniture that you have to keep clean.' The shortcomings of this kind of care had already been recognized and team nursing was introduced on Hamilton when Christine successfully completed an ENB course on 'Nursing the Elderly', to be replaced a few years later by named nursing.

'Named nursing is better because we have less patients to look after and more time to give them. Because older people need time if we want to encourage them to be as independent as they possibly can.'

This is an understatement: the attention and patience required for successful nursing of this kind is phenomenal. To help a patient wash, for instance, can take an hour: 'They can do things for themselves but you have to be with them. You give them a flannel and tell them, "You wash your face;

you do this, and that." And they start washing their face and after a couple of seconds they have lost concentration and stop doing it, and you have got to remind them of what they are doing. You've got to take time.'

And you've got to take that time every day, on every shift. I asked Christine if she found it depressing to work with the same patients over so long a period, knowing that there would be no change in their condition.

'No, I don't mind it, because when you're working with them for so long it is real continuing care that you're giving. You know everything about them and they know everything about you – those that can tell you. But most of them are so confused; and some of them have had a stroke and so they can't talk.'

Other kinds of communication problems also present themselves from time to time. Rani was an Indian lady with no English. She had come to Hamilton from Alf's fifteen months before with some of the same problems as Margaret – obesity, and needing a puréed diet. She couldn't swallow very well and she had a pressure sore on her heel.

Rani had several relatives who came to see her, including a number of children, and they spoke some English, though Christine found them hard to understand. This had created particular problems when the staff began asking Rani's son to buy personal items for her.

This is standard practice on Hamilton, as on other continuing care wards. The NHS provides patients with regulation nightclothes, bedding and towels, with food and medication, but all extras have to be paid for. On Hamilton, 'extras' include soap, orange juice (the ward gets about two bottles a week on the NHS), clothes and special foods like diabetic biscuits. Sometimes the patient's relatives bring in anything that's needed and keep a running check on that patient's personal supplies. In other cases, the pension book is handed over to the ward and the nurses see to it all.

Rani's son, who had been used to handling her pension book at home and counting her pension in with general housekeeping, either could not or would not understand the staff's requests. Part of the problem was that he was uneasy about having his mother in hospital at all; it took Christine some time to win his trust and convince him that she had Rani's interests at heart. She had to work hard to remind him to bring in even the smallest items, like a bar of soap. Christine also thought Rani should have her own quilt, a new dress and a supply of bananas and diabetic biscuits, both of which she had discovered Rani liked. The quilt came, but after a year Rani was still without the other things. Eventually the nurses arranged a meeting with the son, the ward manager, Christine, Rani's social worker and St Wenceslas' finance officer, to lay out the options: either he brought his mother in what she needed, regularly, or else he gave the pension book to the finance officer. He agreed to give them the pension book, and Christine was never sure what the original problem had been, nor what had persuaded him in the end.

Wards like Hamilton simply don't have the resources for interpreters, and communication between non-English speaking patients, their families and nurses relies heavily on the nurses' ingenuity. By the time the pension book arrived, Rani could understand Christine's 'good morning' and repeat it; she would also repeat simple phrases addressed to her, and Christine thought she might have come to understand some basic questions and statements. She had looked forward to giving Rani some treats; now that there was money available for her the first thing she had done was to help her choose a dress from the visiting shop. Unfortunately, Rani never wore it: she died just one week later.

Christine identifies the main components of her work as 'the activities of daily living. You can make them nice, clean and comfortable. Encourage their mobility, those that have difficulty moving and walking. And those that stay in bed all the time and don't have any mobility at all, we prevent them having pressure sores.

'We also look after our clients' spiritual needs. For instance for those who want to go, we get them ready to go to services every Wednesday and Saturday and I arrange for priests, rabbis, etc., to visit them regularly. I also ensure that a priest or rabbi or other person of their spiritual belief sees them when they are very ill.

'And we stimulate them: mental stimulation is one of the big things for the elderly as well.'

When I asked how she provided this, Christine's immediate reaction was to talk me through a kind of timetable. 'In the morning when we look after them [i.e. help them wash and dress, and give them breakfast] I try to do some realistic orientation to stimulate them. Tell them the date first, because if you ask them they would not know; tell them the day, the month and the year. Because although you tell them every day, some of them will still not remember the year the next day. Hopefully some of them will remember when you go back to them in the afternoon.

'Then you tell them the events of the day, the times they are going to have their meal. You ask them, what time do you usually have dinner? That will jog their memories. Then we usually talk about the weather. I might tell them, today it's lovely weather, the sun is shining; what time of year do you think it is? You don't always get the right answer.'

This everyday conversation is as much as the more confused patients can cope with. With others, the nurses may try to arrange trips out of the ward, to different parts of the hospital grounds, or out of the hospital altogether, perhaps to a park. These trips are few and far between: partly because a nurse has to be spared from the ward to take the patient out in a wheelchair, but mainly because the patients are reluctant to go. 'Most of them are not interested in doing anything beyond the ward at all. Some of them will say, "I worked enough when I was younger, now I don't want to do anything. I just want to sit down and do nothing at all." '

Medical wisdom has it that elderly patients should be encouraged to be active; the nurses have to balance encouragement with compassion and respect for the patients' wishes. 'Persuasion is very important for elderly patients. With some people, it is hard to persuade them to do anything; with others it's easier, especially if they take a liking to you. From their point of view, they are doing *you* a favour.'

With very sick patients, little activity is possible beyond eating and drinking. A patient's tastes and preferences then become very important as a source of pleasure and as a means by which nurses can give comfort. They can also be an indication to nurses that a patient's condition is changing. This happened with Lena, in the middle of February.

Lena had been on Hamilton two years. Initially she hadn't wanted to come: she had been nursed once before in St Wenceslas, on a different ward, and had been unhappy there. She and her family had disliked the nurses' attitude. They had agreed to her admission only because there was nowhere else for her to go.

'When she came to us, we already knew from the notes, the nurse-to-nurse communication, that the relatives are very difficult. Even the doctors were getting a bit fed up with this family, saying, "They're always complaining!" She came to us in May the year before last and she died last week. We never had a complaint from the family. The doctors never had a complaint. The patient was a nice, sweet lady; she never complained.'

Lena was frail and diabetic and suffered from Parkinson's Disease; she was also confused at times. She didn't know Christine's name but she recognized her face. Oddly enough, when other nurses talked about Christine, Lena understood who they meant, but she could never remember Christine's name when she was there.

Christine was very fond of Lena. She had also grown close

to Lena's son and daughter-in-law, who came to visit her every day. 'When she first came to us, the son, Dennis, used to call us every morning at 6 o'clock, as soon as he got out of bed, to ask how is his mum. Then the daughter-in-law would come dinner-time and the son would come in the evening. They came like that every day until Dennis got made redundant and the daughter-in-law had to leave work because of illness; since then they come either in the morning or in the evening. They always say to me, "Anything Mum wants, you tell me." '

Lena was not well enough to do very much, and her confusion made her less outgoing than she might have been naturally. Like many of the patients, she had settled tastes: every morning, for instance, Christine would ask her what she wanted for breakfast and every morning Lena would ask for cornflakes without sugar (because she was diabetic), bread and jam and a cup of tea. This menu was unvarying for twenty-two months; then, one morning, Lena had asked for cheese.

Christine had been taken aback. There was no cheese in the ward fridge and she had not brought in any for her own lunch, as she sometimes did. She had apologized to Lena and told her that she would get some for the next day. When Dennis arrived to visit, she passed on the request. He was surprised: Lena had never liked cheese before. However, he brought some in and Lena duly ate it for breakfast the next day – in fact she ate nothing but the cheese.

For a few days, Lena went on eating less of her usual food and taking the cheese. Then one week after the craving had arrived, she said she felt ill. It proved to be the beginning of a rapid deterioration. For a few days, she was up and down. When Christine returned from a day off the next Monday, she noticed a change for the worse. 'I thought she wasn't looking well at all. I asked the nurses if the doctor had seen her today, they said no. I said, "Well, I don't think Lena will last very long. She looks really bad." I said to them, "Can you phone the doctor?" because I was going for a meeting.'

(Doctors do not routinely visit and examine clients on Hamilton every day. They will come if requested by a nurse or if a relative is worried about the person's condition. As Christine put it: 'Remember, Hamilton is our clients' home and at home we call doctors only when we need them.')

The doctor diagnosed bronchial pneumonia. He prescribed antibiotics but Christine was not optimistic; she had seen too many patients on Hamilton die of pneumonia. She gave Dennis and his wife the doctor's diagnosis and tried to prepare them for the likely outcome.

It came quite quickly. When I saw Christine, a week afterwards, it was still very clear in her mind. She seemed to feel a need to relive what had happened. Unprompted, she went on to recount the events of Lena's last twenty-four hours with extraordinary vividness. She spoke concisely, but what she said brought Lena and her bedside immediately alive, probably because they were so clearly still alive to Christine herself.

'I spoke to Dennis on Tuesday evening. Tuesday night with her nightcap Lena vomited. Wednesday when I came on, she had half her breakfast so I asked if she wanted a glass of milk, warm or cold. She said warm. She drank it all.

'Dennis was there. At midday I said to him, "We'll give her only soft soup, nothing else, because I don't think she'll tolerate anything more." He fed her with a spoon. About half past one she vomited. Her granddaughter was there and she's a ward sister: we sat her up and made her comfortable and they went about half past two.

'Then her condition deteriorated. We phoned them – they don't live far away – and asked them if they'd like to come back. Before they reached the hospital, Lena died. She died peacefully. She was comfortable at least.'

Lena's funeral was arranged for the day after our interview and Christine was glad to have been invited. She had been to Margaret's funeral too and found it comforting. It had occurred to her, during these last months, that the other patients and staff on the ward might benefit from some kind of remembrance service. She was now discussing the idea with the ward manager.

'It would have to be on the ward as most of our patients aren't mobile. I got in touch with the chaplain of the hospital and asked if he could come and give the service on the ward and he said, it's a good idea; he'll let me know. I suggested as well that we get in touch with all the people who have lost their loved ones and tell them about our intention.'

There was no date fixed for the service, but Christine thought it probably would happen. It would be the first time, she commented, that the ward had done anything like that. I was surprised – it seemed such a simple, humane idea. I was beginning to grasp the scale of the shortcomings implicit in our approach to elderly care. Hamilton was evidently not a bad ward – Lena had been content there, as she hadn't been elsewhere – yet it had never acknowledged that the patients for whom it was home might want to mourn the deaths of their neighbours.

Working on Hamilton entails facing one constant challenge: how to keep up morale. Patients do not get better and leave; if they leave it is usually because they die. Meanwhile, they are all confused to one degree or another, many of them living in a dislocated world where the present and the past are jumbled. The care the nurses give has no logical progression; for the patients there is no beginning, middle and end, but a series of days and nights which repeat themselves. Each time the nurses come on duty they need to come afresh.

For Christine, striving to give good, all round care was not only a worthwhile effort to make, but a useful means of coping with the down side of nursing the elderly. It gave her something to aim for. It also made her a very good nurse: in the opinion of Mrs Aballa, the head of the continuing care department at St Wenceslas, Christine was as valuable to the ward as the sister, if not more so. (The sister's title, confusingly, was being changed to 'ward manager'.) In fact, Mrs Aballa would have liked Christine to become a sister one day, and for some time now had been encouraging her to do a conversion course to become an RGN.

Christine was undecided. She knew that her role on Hamilton was as support to the ward manager; the senior nursing officer had told her that quite frankly, when she had offered her the transfer there. The ward manager did not like telling people to do things and Christine was asked to back her up in difficult decisions and stand by her. Christine was already shouldering much of a sister's responsibility, so the work held no fears for her. And it would be nice to have recognition, more money and the scope to use her experience and her ideas to greater effect.

Moreover, all the signs were that the NHS would eventually phase out enrolled nurses. It is no longer possible to train as an EN and in many hospitals ENs compete vigorously to get on conversion courses so that they can become registered and improve their employment prospects.

However, the course lasts two years and almost all the studying has to be done in the nurse's own time, while she continues full-time work. Pierre, Christine's husband, was not keen. Her daughter and son (now grown up and living away from home) both thought she should do it and were trying to win him round, but Christine thought it would take a while yet. Meanwhile, the winter months had seen some long-standing problems with her colleagues intensify.

Ever since Christine had been on Hamilton, a few of the other enrolled nurses had been offhand with her. They thought she was too particular and demanded too much of her colleagues. When she was made a team leader, resentment grew and they did not take kindly to her asking them to think up ways in which care could be improved and then set themselves deadlines by which to achieve them.

Christine had grown used to a certain tension in her relations with the other nurses. While she didn't enjoy it, she'd learnt to live with it. This last winter, however, it had become more marked and had begun seriously to wear her down.

Matters came to a head one Tuesday, when her shoes vanished from the cloakroom. As always, she had changed from her own clothes and shoes into her uniform when she came on shift; at the end of the shift, her clothes were still safely in her locker but her shoes, which had been left with everyone else's, had disappeared. She asked the others to help her look for them but there was no sign of them, and in the end she had to give up and go home. The next day, her shoes were back in the place she had left them.

It was a petty little trick and it was the last straw. Christine demanded to know who had taken them and replaced them. No one admitted to it, so she said she would go to management and say she wanted to be moved to a new ward. This prompted one of the other staff members to say that she knew who had taken the shoes. She named a nurse with whom Christine had argued in the past.

This nurse insisted that she had taken the shoes by accident, but Christine told the ward manager that she wanted an apology. So the next day the ward manager held a staff meeting, extracted an apology for Christine and said that this sort of trick was to stop. And rather to Christine's surprise, it did.

She was wary for a few weeks, expecting the cold shouldering to start again, but something fortuitous happened: St Wenceslas instituted a regime of self-assessment among its nurses. They all had to fill out forms which included statements about their personal objectives, listing what they wanted to achieve in the next six months. Christine had already done this kind of thing voluntarily. The nurses who had been hostile to her now needed her guidance, and the murmurings against her died down as the other staff had to seek and accept, more or less graciously, her help.

As spring approached, therefore, Christine was looking forward to a happier time on the ward. She decided that she would enrol in a six-month course of study, starting in October, which would be done largely in her own time. That would give her credits towards her conversion course and might show Pierre that the studying wouldn't necessarily disrupt their home life.

She was also getting to know Edie and Grace, her two new ladies. Christine always referred to her patients as 'ladies' rather than women. I noticed that many of the nurses did this, especially when the patients were elderly: it was a way of signalling respect for them and of acknowledging their right to be addressed on their own terms. ('Ladies' and 'gentlemen' sound quaint to the younger generation; to the elderly they constitute simple good manners.)

As the months went by, Christine was also beginning to speak less of patients and more of 'clients'. This reflected a change in the terminology used at St Wenceslas but it sat very easily with Christine. She liked to call them 'clients', she said; it helped the staff remember that they were nursing individuals who had preferences and rights as well as needs. She and her two new clients were now embarked on the slow, complex process of learning about one another.

Spring

APRIL ON HOWARD, the children's ward, was busy. Kate was well settled in and getting to grips with an influx of surgery cases. March had seen a great rush of tonsilectomies, a seasonal phenomenon which had nothing to do with the weather and everything to do with the fact that the hospital's contracts run from April to April, and there was a backlog of tonsilectomies to perform before the financial year ended. On the bowel disease side, there were many stoma operations scheduled, and the children in for these required intensive nursing. Other children with bowel disorders were coming in for investigative microsurgery, which involved purging their digestive systems beforehand. Kate was now experienced in all these procedures; in fact, she took her turn at explaining them to the students who were arriving on placement.

Kate was much more confident than she had been; she now took in her stride things which had made her nervous in January. Which was just as well, as she was required to take regular turns on the ward's most taxing bay, a group of four boys, three adolescents and an eight-year-old, all in for bowel surgery.

It was an interesting group of patients, both medically and emotionally. Three of the patients (two of fifteen and the eight-year-old) were having iliostomies raised; this is basically the same procedure as a colostomy, but the stoma is raised from the ileum, higher up the alimentary canal than the colon. The other boy, who was sixteen and had Crohn's Disease, was having investigative surgery. He was the focus of some argument: he had an elder sister with bowel disease (it can run in families), who had had a successful stoma operation a few years earlier, and his mother was very keen that he should have the same operation. However, the nature of his disease was slightly different and the doctors felt that an iliostomy wouldn't solve his problems. Although the doctors explained this to the boy and his mother, the mother was reluctant to accept it. It fell to the nurses to try and convince her.

By now, Kate had acquired a good deal of knowledge about bowel disease and stoma operations. She had nursed several children before and after operations and knew what to expect. She had also learnt about the long-term effects of living with a stoma and the psychological problems it can cause.

When first raised, the stoma looks like a tube. This is because, after the diseased section has been removed, the functioning end of the alimentary canal is diverted to an opening made in the abdomen surface, where it is fixed there so that it protrudes an inch or two. It resembles, in Kate's words, 'a sausage'. Later it shrinks right back to the skin and becomes just a hole. Over it the patient wears a sterile, changeable bag, into which waste products flow.

The creation of a stoma and bag is usually a huge relief for young children, because it relieves them of the intense pain caused by their diseased bowel. Once they are used to the bag, they are completely mobile and can do all the things other children do, run, swim, play sports, ride bicycles, activities they have probably been missing out on for years. They can also eat more or less normally, though they should go easy on spicy and salty foods. At this age, freedom from pain vastly outweighs any embarrassment about the bag.

When children reach adolescence, however, problems with body image tend to occur. A mother of a young boy, in for a stoma operation, had recently asked Kate about this. 'I said I honestly didn't know because I'd never met a child *after* the operation. I've only seen them before and while it's being done, when they're still healing and learning about it. But later on I asked sister about it and she told me there's apparently a higher suicide rate after this than after any other operation.'

Since then, Kate had been thinking about the implications of it. She was not so far from adolescence herself and could remember how important it was to feel attractive. With a bag, although you can lead a normal active life, you can't exactly revel in your body. 'You can't wear a tight swimsuit. So many fashions now are governed by wearing tight clothing and how can you do that with a bag that fills up with air and faeces? And they can be smelly if you've eaten something that doesn't agree with you. You have a certain amount of sensation when it comes out, so you know it's happened and can change the bag, but you have no control. Small children aren't very conscious about all this, but fifteen- to sixteen-year-olds are wondering how they'll explain it to a boyfriend or girlfriend.'

Children do receive a certain amount of preparation for what's in store. Specialist nurses known as stoma therapists visit them before they come into hospital. They show them bags, explain how the stoma will work and discuss what life will be like afterwards. There is also a stoma therapist attached to the ward, who visits the children after admission and discusses with them where they would like their stoma to go. The amount of choice they have in this depends on how much of the bowel needs to be removed, but surgeons will do their best to honour the children's wishes.

After the operation, the children are seen by a psychiatrist and a psychologist. Every Monday one of the sisters attends a meeting with doctors, psychiatrist and psychologist, to review the patients' progress. Once they go home, there is usually follow-up help available. 'But in this country it's tricky, because there's a stigma about being seen by a psychiatrist, isn't there?'

The four boys in the bay were very different from one another. Adam, the fifteen-year-old from London, was very quiet before his operation, so quiet that Kate found it hard to get any impression of him and couldn't tell if he was silent through worry or just naturally taciturn. Afterwards, he was rather miserable and demanding – or 'the whinge of the century', to quote Kate exactly. (Kate was inclined to have a robust attitude to adolescents in her care. Just as she had found the teenage tonsilectomy patients exasperating when they refused to eat their cornflakes, she now took a dim view of being asked to do every little thing for Adam. The vagaries of teenagers' behaviour struck a less sympathetic chord in her than they did in Rachel.)

It turned out, however, that much of Adam's lassitude was connected with physical problems. He developed a haematoma (a blood clot) in the remaining section of his bowel and whenever he ate, he vomited. He was put on a drip but he got thinner and thinner, and whenever the nurses tried to start giving him solid food he couldn't take it. Three weeks passed and he continued to lose weight; eventually he was put on TPN (Total Parental Nutrition), as Emma had been. It worked well, giving him nourishment and resting his bowel at the same time. His haematoma went away, he became stronger and, as he felt better, more outgoing.

He began comparing stomas with the other fifteen-year-old, Michael. The two boys had had their operations within a few days of each other, and now they would sit on the edges of their beds, displaying their wounds and discussing them, while eight-year-old Simon, who hadn't had his operation yet, looked on wide-eyed. Adam also discovered that he could tease the nurses by threatening to show his stoma to all the visitors.

'The bags could easily be hidden under pyjamas and bedclothes but the boys liked to show them off. "See how much you've damaged this body! Look at my wound!" I think it was mainly just fun, but the stoma can be uncomfortable at first if it's got things on top of it. It sticks out and it's tender, so in the beginning children tend to have them out. They get used to us coming along and covering it up, saying, "The visitors don't want to see that, show it off between yourselves," because poor old Gran comes in and is faced with this wound!'

This isn't as callous as it sounds. A bad reaction from an unprepared visitor could be very hurtful for the child. As there's no way of ensuring that all visitors are educated and prepared, the nurses opt for some matter-of-fact discretion.

Kate enjoyed nursing the stronger, livelier Adam, although it was sometimes exhausting. When it was time for him to go back on solid food, he fantasized wildly about all the most unhealthy things which he wasn't supposed to eat – pizza, chips, hamburgers – and Kate had to be persistent in making sure he got at least some wholesome food and limiting his intake of junk food.

Michael, the other fifteen-year-old, came in from the West Country with his mother. She had trained as a nurse; Kate could never ascertain whether she had worked after qualifying, but she certainly had a fair amount of knowledge about the general running of the ward. She was staying in Surgery House and was on Howard every day, trying to keep Michael entertained and helping the nurses with the mundane jobs like making beds.

Michael also had problems after his operation, but minor ones. When Kate and the other nurses were cleaning the wound, which had to be done regularly, they noticed that it was infected. 'We couldn't tell if the pus was coming from the edge of the wound or from inside the bowel. The stoma therapist said she thought it was from round the edge and that we had to be really careful as stomas could just drop off on to the floor! So every time we went to clean it we were praying that it wouldn't happen, but we had to "give it a good wiggle" so that if it came off, it would happen here.'

The stoma stayed on, but Michael didn't feel like eating or drinking and he lost a lot of weight and became dehydrated. He was not seriously ill but it delayed his recovery and increased his frustration. He took it out on his mother, telling her to shut up, calling her names and deliberately annoying her by doing his favourite trick – rolling up his eyes so that only the whites showed. 'He looked like something from a horror movie. Because he was so thin and dehydrated he had black eyes and sunken cheeks, and then he'd do this to his mother. She'd sit there, furious, saying, "Don't you *dare* roll your eyes at me!" '

The nurses tried to defuse the tension by making a joke of it in public, but privately they advised Michael's mother to take some time away from the ward and look around London. So she went out, and while she was gone Michael's father telephoned and told Michael in confidence that his elder brother, Sam, had been in a minor car crash and broken his tooth. Michael was told not to tell his mother, as they didn't want to worry her, and Sam arranged to visit Michael and tell him all about it.

Sam duly came a few days later and a farce ensued, whereby the sons chatted aimlessly whenever the mother was around and, as soon as she went away, fell to discussing the accident. Michael wanted to know all the details and was hissing at Sam 'How fast were you going? How did you do it?' Then the mother would come back and want to know why they were whispering. When, eventually, she got the truth out of them, she exploded. She was shouting at them and they were laughing at her; she appealed to the nurses for their opinion; the nurses, knowing from the boys' conversation that not only had Sam been in a crash but that his father had been allowing him licence to do all kinds of things while she was away, were sheepishly amused.

Meanwhile Simon, the eight-year-old, was making a rapid recovery. He had had his operation one week after Michael and Adam, and there had been no complications. Kate was impressed with the way he responded to the nurses: 'He was brilliant. He just got up, moved around, stood up straight, straight away.' One week after his operation, he went home.

His recovery was watched with pleasure by the nurses and with wistfulness by the mother of the fourth patient, John, the sixteen-year-old whose sister had already had an iliostomy. Kate could sympathize with the mother's desire: John was in great pain and had been in and out of hospital repeatedly. The doctors had diagnosed Crohn's and told John and his family that there was no point in giving him a stoma, as the Crohn's might recur higher up in the alimentary canal. He had already been prescribed steroid enemas and washes, but they hadn't worked. Now they were trying Flexical – an all round liquid nutrient rather like TPN, but taken by mouth or by nasogastric tube. Kate found it stomach-turning even to make up.

'It's a milky fluid which smells a bit like baby milk – a real fat smell. And you stand there first thing in the morning, making up pints of it – oh, it's disgusting! John had it through nasogastric tube which is pretty nasty as well – they have to feed the tube up their nose and then swallow it.'

Children take this fluid for six or eight weeks. They start off taking it in hospital, under supervision, then if all goes well they go home and continue with it there. The idea is that it rests the bowel, allowing it time to heal naturally. Unfortunately this wasn't happening with John. Having gone home to continue with the Flexical diet, he was readmitted a few weeks later in great pain.

Exploratory surgery found that he had strictures – narrowing and tightening of the tissue in the bowel. The doctors scheduled him for surgery to split the strictures and relieve the pain. John was now extremely demoralized: he had been having prolonged bouts of severe pain for four years and had been told many times already that various treatments would make him better. Not surprisingly, his mother was more insistent than ever that he should have a bag. The doctors' view, though, was that it would be wrong to carry out such a drastic procedure when there was a strong chance that problems would recur later.

'It's very difficult. Some parents are very accepting that you know what's wrong with their child. Others, like this woman, say, "I've had eighteen years' experience, my eldest child's eighteen, this one's sixteen, I know what's wrong with my child. This worked for my other child, *why* won't you do it for this one?" And of course John just wants the pain to go.'

Having to talk to John's mother, again and again, about why the hospital believed he shouldn't have the operation, made Kate think through the relationship which exists between a child's nurse and the child's parents. The parents of a sick child are often in a panic and, if the illness has been prolonged and the child is suffering, they can come to believe that doctors and nurses simply don't care about their child's pain. The temptation for nurses, then, is to retreat into hospital culture.

'I suppose if I were a parent I'd know what was the matter with my child and I'd know what I wanted done for my child. I'll have to try and remember that when I'm confronted by a parent who does things in a certain way, wants their child spoken to in a certain way. I think part of children's nursing is respecting that. *However,* it's really frustrating when they don't know what's the matter and they're not prepared to listen and change their opinion. They won't let you try to explain.'

In the end, Adam, Michael and Tom had all gone home when John went to theatre to have his strictures cut.

TOWARDS THE END of this busy period, students arrived on the ward. There were five of them, all from the third year of Project 2000, and Rachel Barlow was among them. Rachel was relieved to be coming to Howard: the set had been split into two groups of five for the spring placements, and each group was going to do five weeks on Howard and five on A & E, not at Alf's or the Wavetree, but at a small district hospital further east. Rachel had been dreading going to A & E first; she felt that she simply did not have the experience to cope with emergencies. So she was delighted when she found that she was in the group starting off on Howard.

Apart from the brief 'observation and participation' placements on the CFP, this was Rachel's first real experience on the wards. It was certainly the first time that she was able to get to know a ward in any depth. The students did three shifts a week, of restricted length (7.30 a.m. to 1 p.m. on an early, 1.30–6 p.m. on a late) and were counted as supernumerary. They had certain objectives which they were meant to achieve; for instance, they were supposed to do three theatre visits, following the patients through admission, anaesthetic, operation and recovery.

As ever, Rachel was anxious about her abilities and her lack of experience to date. But she was cheered by her first impressions of Howard, which were good. She liked the range of conditions on the ward: besides the children with bowel disease there were ENT (Ear, Nose and Throat) patients, diabetics, children with eczema and asthma and a couple of children with cancer who were waiting for beds on Walsh, downstairs. She also liked the bright atmosphere and the staff, who were welcoming.

There was no formal assignment of mentors and students (this was often the case, despite college guidelines). Instead, staff nurses would volunteer to explain procedures to students and in some cases, pairings emerged. Often, though, the pairings were tenuous: a staff nurse would go through a student's objectives with her and then scarcely be on duty with her again until the end of the placement. Rachel was to free-float through most of her time on Howard and, due to the way their shifts were arranged, she and Kate were never to be on duty together at all.

For all her lack of confidence, Rachel is an observant person. She watched the nurses on Howard and noticed that there were differences in the way they approached the children. Some seemed better able than others to come at things from the child's point of view. Reading their badges and discovering that some were RGNs and some RSCNs, Rachel realized that she might be seeing the real benefit of the RSCN qualification in action. 'You can definitely tell the difference. It's the way they talk to the children, it's the whole attitude towards them. It's hard to put your finger on it, but they seem more at home with them.'

The first operation Rachel saw was on an eight-year-old Turkish girl, who was having excess cerebral spinal fluid drained off from inside her head. 'She was having a ventrical peritoneal shunt put in. They usually do it when there's too much cerebral spinal fluid, which is causing pressure in the head. They just put a tap like a one-way valve into the head and attach a long thin tube to it. The tube is inserted into the fatty layer just under the skin and runs down along the neck, all the way into the peritoneum [the abdominal cavity]. The fluid drains out through the tube into the abdominal cavity and relieves the pressure.'

Rachel caught up with the little girl, Sevgi, after she had been admitted. From the admission notes she discovered that she had been having lots of headaches and her sight was blurred; her balance was also affected. These were classic symptoms of the condition, which should be cured once the shunt was in place. Rachel could do little to reassure Sevgi but smile at her: neither she nor her mother spoke English, and an uncle had come along to act as translator.

'It was really difficult with her not speaking English, she

didn't know what was going on. Someone had given her a preop chat, but I think the uncle used his better judgement and decided that she didn't need to know the half of it. It's difficult – you've done the research and you know that if children are more fully prepared they do better afterwards, but with him being the uncle, he thought he was doing the best thing.

'It was really sad because she was lying on the table just before they anaesthetized her and her whole body started shaking. She was absolutely terrified and these great big tears were rolling down her face and there was nothing anyone could do. Mum was just standing by her feet, smiling. The poor girl had obviously been absolutely terrified for a long time and nobody had picked up on it.'

The operation itself went well and Rachel found it fascinating. The clinical atmosphere of the theatre and the fact that the patient was covered in green sterile sheets, apart from the area being operated on, made the procedure seem impersonal. The surgeons were assiduous at explaining to the students what they were doing throughout the hour-long operation.

Like Angela when she saw the hysterectomy, Rachel was shocked by the matter-of-fact brutality of the surgeons. 'You know how people often say after an operation, I hurt in a totally different part of my body? Well it's probably because they've had the instruments thrown down on them.'

The insertion of the shunt, however, and its immediate effect, were magical to watch. Sevgi had a huge lump on the back of her head, caused by excess fluid; once the operation was completed, it began to subside. 'Immediately afterwards, within a couple of minutes, you could see it going down. The valve only works if there's so much pressure, though there is a button you can press if you want it to drain fluid anyway. Usually they don't work immediately, but with this one there was so much fluid in there, it just sprang into action. You could watch the lump getting smaller.'

When Sevgi came round after the operation, she was visibly better. Her eyes were brighter and she smiled readily. She was kept in a few days for her progress to be monitored and spent most of the time up and about, playing. By the time she left the nurses had taught her to count up to ten in English.

Apart from admissions and operations, much of Rachel's work consisted of maintaining a safe environment for children (continually shutting doors, checking cot sides, removing potentially dangerous objects). Accident prevention, which they had studied, was put into practice all the time. And, as always, the students were able to spend a lot of time talking to the patients.

The importance of talking took on a new light in the last week of the placement when Rachel arrived for her shift at 1 o'clock and found three-year-old Julie in a bed, very frightened and disoriented, with bruises on her throat. It transpired she had been admitted that morning, after an epileptic fit. The fit had happened at home and her mother had called an ambulance; the staff in Casualty, noticing the bruises, questioned the mother and information began to emerge which, though incomplete, was serious enough to make them call the police and admit the child as an emergency.

Some of the information passed to the sister on Howard went on to the care plan; other parts were confidential, and an air of hushed discretion pervaded all staff discussion of it. Rachel asked various people what was going on and gathered that Julie's mother had become very depressed and tried, unsuccessfully, to suffocate herself. She had then decided to kill Julie first, then herself. Her attempt to strangle Julie brought on the epileptic fit, at which point she had panicked and rushed her to A & E. A & E had called in the police and the mother was now being questioned. However, from what she had said to A & E staff and to the police, it seemed that she herself was the victim of long-term abuse by Julie's father. At handover, Rachel and the other nurses were told that if the father appeared on the ward, they were to phone the police station straight away.

Rachel and a fellow Project 2000 student were assigned to spend time with Julie, talking to her and comforting her. They both felt extremely nervous as they didn't know what to expect. The first thing that struck Rachel was the child's bewilderment. 'She didn't know where she was. She'd been there a good couple of hours and she still didn't know. It hit me that we all assume that because it looks like a hospital and we're in uniform, everyone's going to know where they are. But she didn't have a clue.'

Rachel explained to Julie that this was a hospital and she was being looked after because she hadn't been well. The child was dizzy from the drugs she'd been given and confused. She asked how long she'd be staying, to which Rachel had no ready answer. Then, inevitably, she began asking about her parents. 'She was saying, "Where's my mummy? When can I see my mummy and daddy?" and we didn't know what to say. I went off to find the sister and asked what I should do and she came along and said, "Well, your mummy and daddy aren't very well either. That's why we're looking after you." '

That was the pattern of the afternoon: Rachel and her friend would listen to Julie, talk to her and intermittently hurry off to ask a more senior member of staff for guidance.

'It was so difficult to know how much she was remembering. She was crying and saying, "My neck's hurting" and pointing to where it hurt, but no more than that. I think slowly she's going to be piecing it together.

'All I could think of yesterday was that you never lie to a child because they'll never forget and they won't trust you again if you've lied to them. But I thought, I can't tell her the truth either because I don't know how she's going to take it, whether she's ready to hear, whether she recalls any of it anyway.

'My friend and I had the time to spend with her but a lack of experience in knowing what to say. We kept running off saying, "She's told us so and so, what do we say?" The staff on the ward were really good at suggesting things and helping us.'

I was surprised to learn that the branch programme had so far devoted very little time to the subject of nursing children at risk. Most paediatric nurses are likely to work at some time with abused children or those on the 'At Risk' register. Part of the problem, as Rachel pointed out, is that the whole issue of child abuse has only recently been addressed. 'It's still a new thing for people to deal with. There are so many trains of thought about how to respond: whether you should be really honest about it or whether they're just too young. I think there's a kind of filter system in the mind that shuts things out until they're ready. Maybe in about five years' time it'll come through and they'll start to talk about it, and that to me is when they're ready. You don't want to push it.'

There's also the legal position to consider, should the police want to prosecute. If a nurse has 'led' a child to disclose information, by suggesting that certain things might have happened, then what the child tells her will be considered inadmissible as evidence. Rachel was remembering that as she listened to Julie's anxious questions about her parents.

When I met Rachel to talk about this, it was the morning of the next day. She was very wrapped up in Julie, and feeling a rather guilty mixture of emotions about her. 'It's so tragic. But – it's a horrible thing to say, but it's very interesting. I'm quite looking forward to going in this afternoon and seeing what's happened.'

When Rachel arrived, Julie was still there. Physically she was stronger, though she had a weakness down one side of the body which was almost certainly the result of the fit. Now that the dizzying effects of the drugs had worn off she was bright and friendly, but she was also very anxious and still asking for her mother. So far no one knew whether her mother was to be charged or not and no one had come to visit her, except for a police photographer who had been in that morning to take shots of her injuries in case the police wanted to prosecute. There was anger amongst the nurses today, directed against both the parents, and they were busy trying to find out if a social worker had been appointed, because they wanted to get some clothes for her.

Rachel was still encouraged to talk to Julie, though as she was now on her penultimate day of the placement there were many other things she needed to do to try and round off her experience, not the least of which was to get her report signed by senior members of staff.

It is the responsibility of the qualified staff, including fairly new members like Kate, to write up their views on students who have been on the ward. Kate had not worked with Rachel so couldn't comment on her performance. She had been unofficial mentor to two of Rachel's colleagues, however, which had meant sitting down with them at the start of the placement to help them identify what they wanted to do and trying to keep tabs on them later. She had also helped students learn how to do admissions. She felt that they hadn't been allowed nearly enough time to learn new skills.

'I think it was very unrealistic of the college. They're on for twelve or fifteen days, which is hardly anything, and at the end of that someone's supposed to be competent in, say, admitting a patient. But there are so many skills involved in that, that unless you do one properly every day – I mean I don't feel that confident about admitting them now and I've been doing it for four years. Basically you're supposed to be allowing someone to watch one admission, letting them do it under supervision the next, and then you're assessing them in the one after that to see if they're actually competent. How can they be?

'I wrote on everyone's report that although they had achieved these points, if they had spent much longer they would be much better. I said that they were competent within the limits of their experience and got round it that way. Otherwise you'd have to fail people. I think we all felt this was a problem. They had a lot of theory but the practicality of sitting down with people and communicating with them is really hard.'

Rachel got her report signed and the next day she finished on Howard for the time being. When she returned, in the summer, she would be on rostered service, pitching in with the registered nurses on unsocial hours and night duty. Before she left she said goodbye to Julie, who was still there, in borrowed clothes.

O N THE WESTERN edge of the Alf's site, about as far from Howard as it could be, is Marlowe AIDS ward. Its décor is soothing greys and pale blues and there is none of the volubility that characterizes Howard on a typical day. Yet Marlowe and Howard have one thing in common: they are both well resourced and their contrasting styles are deliberate, not forced on either through necessity.

AIDS is currently a well-funded area of medicine. Seen as a high priority by the government, it receives grants as well as a generous allocation of NHS funding. Charities raise money for wards and hospices; companies and individuals make contributions. 'We're on a par with children's wards for receiving charity,' according to Sister Liz Howlett. 'Money isn't a problem for us at the moment. I wish it could be the same for everyone.'

Marlowe is an eight-bed ward, built at the beginning of the 1990s. Together with the GU (Genito-urinary) clinic at

Alf's, and the GU clinic at Wavetree, it makes up the St Alphege's HIV/AIDS unit. (The GU clinics see patients with other conditions too, but HIV-related work is an increasing part of their remit.)

Marlowe is tucked away in a corner of Alf's, with no sign pointing to it other than one which reads 'Genito-Urinary Medicine'. Along a blank corridor and up a flight of stairs, a pair of double doors bears the name of the ward and a handwritten notice saying 'This is NOT the Day Clinic'. It all seems rather anxiously discreet.

Inside, the unit consists of an L-shaped corridor with a small staff room, some cupboards and a tiny kitchen to the left, then a square day area. The nurses' station is opposite this, in the turn of the 'L'. Leading off the other, longer arm of the corridor are eight individual rooms.

Depending on the severity of their illness, patients on Marlowe might stay in bed, go into the day room or even go out of the hospital for a couple of hours at a time. The atmosphere on the ward is fairly relaxed and friends, relatives and partners of the patients come and go at will, often bringing in food and heating it up in the kitchen microwave. People on Marlowe are ill, however, and a kind of hush pervades the corridor.

The day area is used in a low-key way, usually by one or two people at a time. It doesn't exactly lend itself to parties, being furnished in office-reception style with armchairs, a television, a stack of videos, electronic scales and two tall bookcases carrying the entire range of Penguin classics in paperback (a donation from the publishers). 'No one ever seems to read them,' Liz remarked when she was showing me round.

Nurses who now have several years' experience in HIV and AIDS seem to fall into two categories: those, often men, who came to it with a good knowledge of the issues surrounding HIV and sometimes with a background of involvement in voluntary counselling or buddying work, and those who became involved more or less accidentally when HIV and AIDS units were starting up. Liz is one of the latter.

It took me a little while to sort out a coherent impression of Liz. She is in her early thirties, very quietly spoken, and talks about her work in concrete terms: about giving people choices in their treatment, about pain relief, about the reaction of their families and partners to their illness. At first I thought that she wasn't particularly interested in the political and social issues surrounding AIDS but gradually I realized that I was mistaken. She is, quite deeply, engaged with these but she addresses them through her work, where they regularly affect her patients' lives.

Moreover, I was coming at the subject of AIDS nursing with a very one-sided awareness of the issues, principally as they affected gay men. But increasingly, the patients on Marlowe include African Caribbean people: AIDS is widespread in several African countries and there is a large African Caribbean immigrant population in Wavetree. The issues which arise in these cases are quite different and not so widely discussed. Liz was recognizing and exploring them as they confronted her.

In fact, Liz is profoundly interested in questions of social control and the principle of individual freedom and responsibility. She is also perplexed by the question of how to die: at almost every meeting we had, she would talk about the dilemma that faces people who learn that they have only a short time to live.

Liz decided to become a nurse when she was eighteen, after a year working as a secretary in her home town in the south of England had left her bored and restless. Her father, mother and sister were all nurses, so the profession was respected in the family. Nevertheless, her parents were not overjoyed at her choice: 'They thought I'd have a better life if I did something else.'

Liz did her RGN training at the start of the 1980s, outside London, and failed the exams. 'In those days there were two exams at the end of the three years and you had three chances to get them. I failed three times. Looking back now, I'm not surprised. The practical side was no problem, but I didn't have any real grasp of what it was I was doing. I think I was too young.'

She had done well enough to become an enrolled nurse, so she worked for two years in various wards, including Casualty and ITU (Intensive Therapy Unit), before coming to London with a friend who was also a nurse and doing agency work. 'We did it for about a year altogether. At first we lived in bed and breakfasts, then we got a flat. It was OK, we quite enjoyed it. There was no pressure other than to work a lot to pay the bills. But if we disliked a job, we didn't have to go back.'

By now it was the second half of the 1980s and public awareness of AIDS was not so much growing as exploding. HIV and AIDS wards were beginning to evolve at certain hospitals, and Liz began a long stint of nights on one such ward at a big hospital in west London. She enjoyed the work and liked the other staff, so she applied for and got a permanent post as an enrolled nurse.

Liz remained there for five years. She did a six-month refresher course of RGN studies (mostly in her own time) and this time passed the exams. As an RGN, she learnt about HIV and AIDS as the other medical staff learnt, and took what specialist courses came her way. She built up close relationships with the other staff and with the long-term patients who would be admitted with an AIDS-related disease, have it treated successfully and return home until next time.

At the end of five years, however, the professor in charge of the ward was offered the post of heading the new HIV/AIDS unit at St Alphege's. When he decided to move, several of the staff opted to go with him. Alf's advertised a sister's job on the new Marlowe Ward; Liz applied and got it.

Liz had come to Marlowe, therefore, as one of the founding staff. They had brought with them a few of the patients from the west London hospital as well, but on the whole the intake of Marlowe's was drawn from the St Alphege's and Wavetree Health Authority.

'I do notice a big difference in the kinds of patients coming in. In west London we were seeing predominantly middle class – what do you call it, social class two? – gay men, quite well off, artistic. Here it's a greater mix: the majority are still gay men but there's a higher percentage of women. They tend to be working class and they include African women and some drug users; a lot of them have families.'

On Marlowe Ward, Liz sees people in all stages of HIV and AIDS. Definitions of when HIV becomes AIDS do not seem to be very firmly fixed; basically, people who have tested positive for the virus are said to have HIV or to be HIV (I never heard a nurse or doctor on Marlowe say 'HIV positive'). Someone with HIV might be perfectly healthy or might have relatively minor symptoms like a difficulty in retaining weight or getting over colds. (Because the virus attacks the immune system, people with HIV have to be extremely careful about exposing themselves to everyday infections.)

In the long term, however, people with HIV are known to be susceptible to certain diseases. These include TB, pneumonia and certain forms of cancer, particularly Kaposi's Sarcoma (a skin tumour) and lymphoma (which can involve tumours of the brain and internal organs and precipitate paralysis and personality disorders). Certain viruses are commonly associated with HIV, notably cytomegalovirus (CMV) which can cause blindness. Some of these are curable, others can be treated so that they go into remission, but if you have HIV, each bout of illness weakens you and although you may recover well and look very fit, your body will be less able to resist the next illness.

In the HIV/AIDS field, these illnesses are known as 'AIDS-related' or as 'opportunistic infections'. Broadly speaking, once someone with HIV contracts one or more of these diseases, he or she can be considered to have AIDS. But nurses and patients alike are sensitive to the nuances of language and very often they continue to use the phrase HIV as a matter of preference. After all, each disease has its own symptoms and effects and requires its own treatment: someone with Kaposi's Sarcoma is not experiencing the same thing as someone with CMV. And someone who has recovered from pneumonia and is up and about and back at work is actually free of disease for the time being, despite the underlying HIV condition.

In early spring, as Marlowe Ward approached its second birthday, all eight beds were full as usual. Since opening, it had worked to capacity and for some time now the HIV unit had funded an additional two beds on a neighbouring Alf's immunology ward as an overflow. Next year Marlowe looked set to expand further: the unit had plans to take over the majority of beds on a brand new twenty-bed infection control and immunology ward. Construction would be starting on the Alf's site this coming autumn – if, of course, the hospital survived.

The staff on Marlowe were fairly optimistic about the future. As one of Alf's leading specialities, they felt that the unit would survive in some form, even if it had to transfer to a different site. But in any case, thoughts of the future took second place in Liz's mind at the moment, behind the immediate demands of the workload.

Patients on Marlowe are shared among two teams of nurses, but as ever with this arrangement there is a good deal of crossover. Liz heads one team, Peter, a charge nurse, the other. Their jobs involve some hands-on care of the patients and (rather more) supervising and co-ordinating of the day-to-day running of the ward.

Nursing AIDS patients is not very different from nursing any seriously ill person. The infections usually require aggressive drug therapy during which the patient's condition must be monitored very closely, so that drugs can be adjusted and any other developing conditions picked up and treated. Observations are very important, therefore, and if a patient is on an intravenous drip, nurses will also check the machines every few hours. Marlowe's machines are computerized, with digital displays and bleeps to alert the staff if anything jams or runs low.

Nurses also help patients cope with side effects of the drugs, nausea or dizziness for instance, and with some of the more distressing symptoms of AIDS, such as the violent diarrhoea that often afflicts people as their immune systems deteriorate. This is where basic, old-fashioned care comes in: the nurses may be using sophisticated equipment and have a high level of specialist knowledge but they also need to keep the patients clean and comfortable.

The precautions taken against cross-infection are the same as on any other ward. Wherever you work in a hospital, you are supposed to wear gloves when coming into contact with body fluids, to dispose of used needles, scalpels and dressings immediately and safely, and to keep equipment and utensils sterile.

The amount of this kind of work Liz does depends on how busy the ward is. When a few extremely sick patients are in, crises can occur and then everyone does what's necessary. This apart, she generally gets closely involved with the patients on her team, talking over their prognosis and discussing the various forms of therapy, usually drug therapy, open to them.

'Informed consent for the patients means knowing what they're taking, what the results are and what the possible side effects may be. Our patients are very clued up – it's murder! It's good in one way: you don't need to explain the illnesses and drugs in minute detail and simplistic terms, as they already know about them. It keeps the staff on their toes – sometimes patients will have read about things we haven't come across. And the patients can contribute to their own treatment and feel more in control.

'Patients will sometimes refuse drugs. We are trained to respond to patients' choices, to say, "Well, there's this alternative. We feel it might not be as good for *you* but if you prefer it we'll try it as a compromise." '

She also gets to know patients' families and partners well. Often patients will be preparing to leave Marlowe and return home, and the people close to them need to be knowledgeable about their condition and the drugs they are taking. If patients are going home alone, then Liz will discuss with them the need for support services, and work with the community and social workers attached to Marlowe to try and get the patients what they need.

So far this year had been busy in a measured way. Each bed had been occupied all the time, but the majority of the patients were stable and the nurses had been able to pace themselves. In March, however, there had been an influx of extremely sick patients who required a high level of active care. Some of them Liz knew well from previous admissions; others were new.

Bernard, a thirty-one-year-old man, was one of the new ones. He had been admitted at the end of March. He had tested positive with HIV eighteen months earlier, but had been in good health until January of this year, when he'd begun to feel ill with a cold. The cold had turned into infected sinuses and he now felt generally unwell. The symptoms did not seem to point to anything specific and so he was in for investigations.

Then there was David, aged thirty-two. By contrast, Liz had known him for two years, ever since he had first been diagnosed with HIV; he was one of the patients who had followed the staff from west London. So far David had been lucky. He took good care of himself and had been attending the clinic regularly for check ups, and nothing had been wrong. Now, though, a tumour had been discovered in his chest and he was staying on Marlowe for a couple of weeks to have it graded. This involved several investigative procedures. When the results finally came, they were not good; he had a very aggressive form of lymphoma. Treatment would involve several months of chemotherapy and the drugs used produced very unpleasant reactions. And, as Liz said bleakly, 'At the end of that he probably won't have much time left'.

David's prognosis was a terrible shock for David himself, who still felt quite well. His partner was stunned too and even the staff were shaken. Liz was still feeling her way round the emotional impact of it when we spoke: 'It's very difficult to believe, even for us, when a healthy person comes down with a very aggressive condition like that. At thirty-two, you expect another thirty years of life. What do you do? I can't imagine what I'd do if it happened to me. Probably carry on as normal. What else could you do? I know some people say they'd spend up on their credit cards or go on a big holiday, but to me that's like stopping being yourself. But then, you can't go on doing everything, you're not physically able to. David's carried on working, right up to the diagnosis, but he'll stop now.'

Although David's condition was very serious, he was not going to stay in hospital indefinitely. His course of chemotherapy would involve his receiving large doses of drugs intravenously, at intervals of a few weeks. As he had cancer, he could be treated either on Marlowe or on Preston, the oncology (cancer) ward: he would probably be going on to both at different times, according to bed availability. David's course would begin at once. In preparation, he had a Hickman line inserted.

On Marlowe, one hears frequent references to Hickman

lines. They are plastic tubes which are surgically implanted into the patient (usually into the chest), with one end feeding into a vein and the other extruding from the body. Intravenous drugs can then be administered through the tube and when it isn't in use it can be capped off.

Hickman lines are widely used for cancer patients receiving chemotherapy. They are convenient, being semi-permanent; they minimize the discomfort involved (the patient cannot feel the drug going in) and they are relatively simple to use, so that if a patient's condition is stable, he or she may be able to receive the chemotherapy at home.

For the same reasons, many AIDS patients have Hickman lines. Because of their weakened immune systems, people with AIDS-related conditions often need regular doses of intravenous drugs. These drugs tend to be toxic, which means they have severe side effects, so frequent monitoring is necessary, but at least with a Hickman line the patient can leave hospital and go home.

This independence is enormously important to people with AIDS, who have lost control over their lives in so many other ways. It is also important to the hospital in purely practical terms, freeing beds for other patients. Then there is the fact, in Liz's experience undeniable if unquantifiable, that people often improve after getting home.

'I've known people say that the treatment is making them feel worse than the infection. They go home and come back a month later looking really good and saying, "Told you so!" It happens quite often. I think it's partly that they go back to their own environment, they have the food they like, their spirit rallies and their fight comes back. Lying in a hospital bed can make you very depressed and disempowered.'

David was eager to go home. He was shocked by what was happening to him and wanted to return to some kind of normality as soon as possible. During the last week of his stay on Marlowe, Liz spent a lot of time talking to him and his partner, Gordon, about the care he would need at home. She also helped teach them how to use the Hickman line: although David was to come back into hospital for his chemotherapy, there might be other drugs that would eventually be administered at home, through the Hickman line. In any case, they needed to know how to look after it and keep it clean. Liz showed them how to flush it out with saline to keep it sterile, how to screw on the specially designed drugs bottles and how to cap it off.

As David left, another familiar patient was coming back in. Amal, a Sudanese woman, had spent weeks on the ward before Christmas for treatment of retinitis, the eye disease caused by CMV. Untreated, it causes blindness; two different drugs which control it are available, but they are highly toxic, with unpleasant side effects, and patients must take them two or three times a week for the rest of their lives.

'She stayed in to have the treatment and was really ill. She got fevers, which we couldn't find a reason for. And the drugs gave her nausea, with vomiting. They made her feel terrible, so in the end she decided to stop them and she went home, knowing that she'd probably lose her eyesight. She just couldn't cope with the way the drugs made her feel. She was at the end of her tether after being in so long and she has a little girl she wanted to get back to.

'Then a few weeks ago her eyesight deteriorated and she went almost blind in one eye and so she's decided to start treatment again. I think you can't quite believe it's going to happen to you until it does. But she's in again now and it looks like the condition won't get any worse. She'll have to stay on the drug though, and it is horrible. Apart from nausea and vomiting, a major side effect is renal failure and people can die of that if it's not picked up fast.'

For the time being, however, Amal felt strong enough to endure the treatment and to undergo further tests. When she had left hospital last time, she had abandoned investigations into her fevers. She hadn't been able to face being pulled around any more and she'd been worried about her daughter. Now, a cousin of hers had come over from Sudan and was taking care of her child, so she asked Liz for a meeting with the registrar and they arranged for a series of tests to start at once. They would take ten days to complete – a gruelling experience but at least at the end of it the doctors might know what was causing the fevers and be able to prescribe something.

If it was heartening to see that Amal was responding to treatment, it was proving very different with Bernard. Since he had been admitted, his condition had deteriorated steadily. The doctors could find nothing major wrong with him, but he had a number of minor infections and as soon as one was cleared up, another one would get worse, and new ones would develop. A common problem with AIDS-related infections is that the drugs that treat one kind of infection may actually predispose the patient to getting another: Bernard was unlucky and his treatment turned into a vicious cycle. By the end of April, he had lost a great deal of weight and was extremely weak and depressed.

Because she felt powerless to help him, Liz found Bernard's decline quite hard to bear. 'Nothing's going right for him, it's becoming a series of disasters. The diagnosis is the main problem because it's multiple – one thing gets treatment and the treatment causes something else, or something else that's lurking there gets worse. It's so frustrating. You get one good day and think, oh, something good's started to happen! Then the next, you're back to square one. And we just don't really know why he's so sick. I think all the nurses have got a feeling of uselessness, inadequacy.'

Bernard got no better. Throughout May he grew weaker and sicker, until he was completely dependent. There was still no clear diagnosis, but it was obvious that he wasn't going to live long. In the end, the staff told him that there was nothing else they could do for him. By this time, Bernard was drifting in and out of consciousness and communication was limited. His partner, John, and his family, who had been in regular attendance at the hospital, told Liz and the other members of staff that they were going to take him home.

'Personally I was glad, because he was going to die within a few days and it was so much nicer for him. So his partner took him home and he died the next day. The family came to see us afterwards and said he'd opened his eyes and recognized everything around him, in his own bed and his room. But it was such a terrible illness.'

For Liz, Bernard's death was the worst thing about April and May. Several weeks later, her voice still tailed off when she talked about him, and she referred to Bernard now and again as 'the young guy', although in fact he was the same age as many of her patients.

The second worst thing about May was a much older patient, who placed a different kind of strain on the staff, one which at times contained elements of black farce.

Edward was in his sixties, married with four children. He was admitted with Kaposi's Sarcoma, very sick and very confused. (A form of dementia is sometimes associated with AIDS.) From the outset, it was obvious that relations within the family were complicated. 'There was a confusion about his records, and it turned out he'd been leading a double life. He had gay friends and gay relationships, but he hadn't talked about it to his family. He'd actually been in before, but under another name.

'When he came in this time, some members of the family knew and others didn't. The wife knew that he had gay friends and that he had HIV – I think she'd only found out recently – and she was *furious* and didn't want to talk about it. She didn't really want to know any details. Most of the older children knew but the youngest daughter, who was eighteen and still at school, didn't.'

The staff could discuss the true nature of Edward's illness

with his eldest children and with his wife, on her rare and reluctant visits. But they had to remember to refer to it only as skin cancer when the youngest daughter was around.

Added to this was the fact that Edward was still using two names; his gay friends were arriving and asking for him by the name he had used on his previous admission. The staff had a terrible time trying to remember who was able to meet whom. The youngest daughter wasn't supposed to meet the friends; moreover, Edward's wife made it clear that she wanted no contact with them either. She would usually let the staff know when she was planning to come in, and Edward would engineer it so that his gay friends stayed away then.

Liz's problem (apart from simply trying to keep track of people) was that Edward's wife didn't want to learn anything about his condition. Yet if and when Edward returned home, he would take a lot of looking after. The one saving grace of the situation was the elder daughter: 'She knew everything and she was brilliant. She works quite close by and she came in every day at lunchtime and tried to organize the whole of the family to act as go-between for the parents.

'I talked to her a lot and she was very strong that the youngest girl shouldn't be told. She was doing her exams and the family was terrified it would throw her off. And she told me that when she was younger a favourite uncle of hers had died and years after, they'd told her he'd committed suicide and she was furious at them for telling her. Because she'd always remembered him as this lovely uncle and it affected all her memories. So she felt it wasn't a good idea to tell her sister ... but I think the sister must have known. At eighteen these days – at least there must have been some pretty big question marks.'

The subterfuge went on for weeks, while Edward continued to be very sick. Through the eldest daughter, Liz managed to impart a certain amount of information to the wife and, rather against Liz's better judgement, the youngest daughter went on believing that her father simply had cancer.

'At times this last month has been, "Aaagh! Whatever's going to happen next?" But looking back you can see the funny side. Every so often you're running round flapping and then you think: "Well, what's the worst that can happen?" We often get these situations where someone doesn't want other people to know certain things and usually in the end someone makes a mistake, or the people guess and come straight out with it.'

Before that could happen, Edward began to respond to treatment. He stabilized and reached a stage where Marlowe wasn't the right place for him. He'd had the intensive treatment they could offer and should now move on. His improvement was quite marked; he was also much less confused and, in his own words, 'walking and talking like a normal person'. A bed was found for him in a different unit and he went, one Tuesday afternoon.

The next day a phone call came through to Marlowe: it was the new unit, to say that Edward had died in his sleep, quite unexpectedly and apparently of a heart attack. Liz could hardly believe it: 'It's just so ironic. We've all been walking round with our mouths open! We've had all this complicated deception going on all month, and then he goes and dies of something that has nothing to do with cancer or AIDS!'

O VER IN A & E, spring had arrived in a flurry of administrative activity, making heavy demands on Janet Moore. Several sets of students were on placement in the department: seven from the degree course, four from the RGN course and three from an enrolled nurse (EN) conversion course. They were staying in the department varying lengths of time, but while they were there, it was Janet's responsibility to see that they got the practical experience they needed.

'This all actually makes more work for us. We've physically got more bodies about and people say, "Oh, you've got loads of nurses here," but the degree course girls and the conversion course nurses are all supernumerary, so they shouldn't officially be counted in the numbers. But I do count them in, otherwise you'd have so many people here, plus agency, it would just be a farce.

'The degree course girls quite enjoy doing hands-on nursing: I tell them to go and attach themselves to someone and they have the benefit of being able to see things as and when they're happening. You can say, "Go and watch this down in resus; go and see this in ops. There's something interesting going on, go and observe it." It's quite nice. But the strain is on you because academically they're very bright but clinically their knowledge isn't as broad as, say, the RGN students who are coming through, because they don't have continuous clinical exposure. Their last placement would have been about six months ago.'

Janet arranged the duty rosters so that there was a mix of different types of student on each shift. They seemed to get along well together and she was amused to observe that they all had one thing in common: 'They're all terrified of coming down here! They're worried about what they might be asked to do and that's uniform, even for the conversion course nurses who are qualified and have been for some time. Because this isn't their area of expertise they can be worried sick and some of them walk round with faces as white as sheets.'

Janet had in the past done some formal teaching, but this time when the college requested a one and a half hour lecture, they left her only two days to prepare, so she refused. 'But if something comes up down on the department, I'll teach them there. I do very little teaching now because my time is all taken up here. I do department-based teaching: we had a session this morning on how to put slings on.

People always get in a complete knicker knot with those. They don't know where to put the knots or the flaps – and there's always four or five ways to put a high sling on the shoulder. It's very basic stuff. You're continuously teaching anyway. If something interesting comes in you'll be saying to them: "Now why am I looking at this side? Why did I find this? What would you be looking for in a urine sample now?" You can do it without even thinking about it.

'I love teaching, I adore it, but I wouldn't want to do it full time. It's nice to teach out of the department and students enjoy being with someone who's teaching anecdotally, out of expertise, because they then start to see a person rather than a bunch of symptoms. You may be able to tell an anecdote about someone and describe them physically, as a person, and that will stick in their minds much more.'

Besides the students, there were many other changes on the staffing front. Eight nurses had left the department in the last few months: four to go on a certificate or diploma level A & E course, three for other hospitals and one to the Wavetree. Six junior nurses had been taken on to replace them and Janet was busy shortlisting applicants for interview for two more senior posts.

Most of the staff moves, Janet thought, had been natural career developments, but she conceded that a sense of insecurity was beginning to creep in to the department. The regional health authority responsible for Alf's area had just announced, in a consultation document, that it did not consider Alf's A & E vital to emergency services in the region. In other words, it would support the government if it decided to close the department down or turn it into an office-hours only minor injuries unit.

This was a severe blow to A & E. It also had ominous implications for the survival of Alf's as a whole, because most of the 'active' (hospital jargon for unplanned) admissions came through A & E. I was amazed to hear this, but Janet explained: it was not that Alf's had a high incidence of patients who fell ill suddenly or through injury; it was because some local GPs were routinely using Alf's A & E as a diagnosis clinic for patients who were ill and might need hospital treatment.

'Most GPs here don't know their backsides from their elbow. I've been looking at how many patients were admitted through a GP referral. The ones I've taken were those whose GPs had bothered to contact a relevant speciality and say, "This patient needs admission." The figures are quite interesting. Last month less than 25 per cent of patients were admitted into hospital that way. The rest, over 75 per cent, came through A & E.'

She showed me the figures for the current month, which she was just calculating: they told the same story. Of a total 449 admissions, just 136 were GP referrals to specialities; A & E had dealt with the remaining 313. And many of those 313 had arrived in A & E clutching letters from their GPs, 'with requests that we look at them and – "Do the needful" is the phrase they like to use.'

Janet acknowledged that some GPs might be sending patients via A & E as a deliberate tactic to bypass waiting lists and get them in as emergency admissions. But she felt that others were simply trying to get A & E to do their work for them. For fund-holding GPs, emergency admissions may also be financially advantageous, as they are excluded from the contracts between GPs and hospitals, i.e. they are free to the GPs (the health authority usually pays).

This was was not only a misuse of A & E; it meant that, now the department was threatened, the whole hospital was vulnerable. Unless local GPs changed their approach to referrals overnight, the closure of A & E would lead to an immediate and possibly massive fall in Alf's admissions. In time, local GPs might well learn to 'do the needful' themselves and refer their patients to Alf's individual specialities; in the short term, however, they were far more likely simply to refer them to the A & E departments of other hospitals. The patients might eventually be admitted to Alf's, if their health authority or GP had contracted to buy services there or if there were bed shortages at other hospitals, but there would inevitably be a period when Alf's was admitting fewer active patients. These figures would support the government's case against Alf's.

As the implications sank in, I was surprised that staff all over the hospital were not talking about them and that the Save Alf's campaign wasn't making a big issue of them. But in fact it was a sign of something I would be quite used to before the year ended: the self-contained character of the various directorates within the hospital. The loyalty of nurses was to their ward and their department; they would know how that worked within the directorate, but they seemed to have little sense of how the different parts of the hospital fitted together, or of how a change in one might affect all the others.

Janet did not appear remotely surprised, but she was angrier than at our last meeting. She'd heard that the hospital with which Alf's was supposed to merge (call it 'the Thames Hospital') was proposing that Alf's become the 'cold' end of the district, receiving only expected admissions, planned surgical procedures, etc. 'Thanks a bunch!'

She was scornful at the prospect of the local population being sent back to GPs in whom they had no faith and predicted that if A & E did become a minor injuries unit, they would end up doing as much 'needful' as ever. But ultimately, she didn't quite seem to believe in any of it.

In April, she went to a large and rowdy meeting of senior A & E nurses throughout the region. A & E consultants were there too and a representative from the Patients' Charter Group. There was one proposal in the charter which was of great concern to the A & E departments: assessment of patients within five minutes of their arrival.

This 'target', to use charter jargon, had been identified

months ago as desirable for all hospitals' A & E departments. The board of directors at Alf's was urging Janet and her staff to achieve it, in the hope that this would count in their favour and help save the hospital. But the A & E staff at Alf's and in most other hospitals were vigorously resisting. Their objection was that assessment time cannot be reduced to a notional figure which applies equally to all patients. Some conditions require immediate care and if they are to receive it, then patients with less urgent conditions, the sprained wrists and cut fingers, must wait.

'If it's something like abdominal pain, it could be anything from a bit of wind or constipation to a ruptured ectopic pregnancy. That patient needs to be properly triaged: you sit them down, take a history from them; you ask them if they're on medication – that can make an awful lot of difference – if they've got any allergies. You can do things like test the urine – in something like abdominal pain in a woman who might be pregnant, the finding can change the priorities quite dramatically.

'And you have to give first aid to a lot of patients. If you've got someone with an arterial bleed from a laceration, you need to see to it sooner rather than later. You need to apply pressure, you may need to lay them flat, you need to give them a bit of *care*, which you can do with triage.

'What if three or four patients turn up at once? I might have someone with a chest pain out there and I need to take him to the resuscitation room. Now I'm not going to say, "You walk in there by yourself and I'll call through" so that I can get on with assessing the others. I'm going to take him down there myself and make sure he's safe, hand him over to the nurse, pass on what he's told me. This is a fairly typical government directive which takes no account of the human element.'

All this and more was said at the meeting. Tempers were running high amongst the senior nurses and the representative from the Patients' Charter Group had a rough ride. 'It was like Daniel going into the lions' den! A & E senior nurses, as a group, are not quiet people at the best of times and the consultants can be even worse. There was absolute support in saying, "This is a load of rubbish. Why do you want us to implement it?" It was very comforting to see such a united front from the consultants because they're rather lone persons. It was very cheering. But I don't know if any ground was gained. At the end of the day this is still what they want us to do.'

The other big event in A & E took place on a weekend. Early on a Saturday morning, when the department was quiet, a telephone call came through for one of the nurses. It was her fiancé, a policeman: he told her, unofficially, that the police had received warning of a large bomb in the commercial district near Alf's. The hospital was likely to be put on standby.

Janet was on duty at the time, one of the skeleton staff that keeps Alf's Casualty going at weekends. No one in the department took the news very seriously; hoax warnings happen all the time. Then the phone rang again, and this time it was an official police call, putting them on standby.

'We thought, "Hmmm . . ." We've never had a major incident at the weekend before. We were a bit thin on the ground really, but thankfully we were all regular staff.'

There is a prescribed procedure for major incidents (m.i.'s in hospital speak). Patients were cleared from the treatment areas; those waiting for treatment were asked to go to a hospital in the opposite direction from the commercial district. Ambulances bringing patients in were diverted to those hospitals too. Off-duty medical staff were alerted in case back up was needed.

'The trouble was, I had *so* many people ringing up saying, "Do you want me to come in?" I wished they'd stop because I was trying to get on with emptying the department. We did get it clear. Then we were here waiting. We knew the bomb was supposed to go off at 10.20.

'Ten twenty-seven the bomb went off and we felt it because it was only half a mile down the road. I was standing under a light fitting and all the dust shook out on to my head. I said, "Oh, that was a bit loud." But we were all quite confident that nobody would be hurt because it was on a Saturday, in a business street, with a lot of warning. We thought the offices would all be empty. We were wrong. They'd all come in on their flexitime, hadn't they?'

The street hadn't been evacuated fully when the bomb went off and people were injured by flying debris. Then news came that some people were trapped in basements, where they had gone for safety.

'Patients began coming in, cut by glass from the blown out windows. We saw a total of thirty-one or thirty-two. It was one of the longest standbys we've ever done. We were on for six and a half hours which is very unusual, but that was because all those people were trapped and we didn't know what condition they were in. We didn't know how secure the basements were. We thought we might have had lots of multiple injuries; people could have been having panic and asthma attacks down there. There was a spate of people with cuts coming through, and lots of doctors, and we were seeing people so quickly that we cleared them all. We kept thinking, "There's going to be loads more, keep going . . ." and there weren't. There was one fatality, he was found quite late on in the afternoon.'

Five of the patients were admitted. Janet felt they were probably being over-cautious with some of them, but the staff were wary of letting people go home and having them collapse with shock. 'With the psychological effects of something like that, you can never tell. They had suffered lots and lots of cuts from bits of flying glass, but they were incredibly calm. I don't know if it was just the sense of relief at being taken out of it all. Perhaps it's the sense of being on the edge and then someone pulling you back from it into safety. They were very, very quiet. There wasn't even anger expressed.'

During the following week, there was a steady flow of people coming in who were suffering in some way or other from the after effects of the bomb. Some had been thrown back by the blast and were hurt when they fell; many were temporarily deaf. Emotionally, they seemed more vulnerable than those who had been in on Saturday. 'In some ways I think they suffered because they hadn't come through the hospital system then and hadn't been recognized as victims of the bomb. Days later I spoke to a lad who said, "I can't believe it. I walked past that building not five minutes before it went off and no police cordon stopped me. I turned around and saw the front of the building blow out. I just can't believe it." He was still stunned and in a way he needed his own form of therapy, and because I'd been on duty it was as if I'd been through it too because I'd received everyone. It was like a purging of that episode for him.'

One week after the bomb, the department ran a follow-up clinic for the patients involved. This is common practice these days, ever since the Kings Cross fire in the 1980s made the need known. Alf's, because of its central location, has since then dealt with many m.i.'s and the department has learnt from each one.

'Some of the patients who came needed stitches taking out but mostly it was to see how they were getting on and if anyone needed to be referred for stress debriefing or stuff like that.

'Most of them were dealing very well with it. Some of them had been to their GPs who'd been less than helpful. They praised the help lines which had been set up, with trained counsellors. We'd also referred some to the hospital's counselling service.

'A couple of people were picked out who needed specific

counselling. That might go on over several weeks; we try to get them to see the same person again and again so they have continuity. But you don't actually have to be a trained psychiatrist to sit down and talk about a lot of this – patients just need a point of contact. They'll often get that here, going to one of the specific clinics for whatever their injury is. It's medical follow up but they see it as a form of therapy as well.'

All the staff had been offered stress counselling too. However, none of them felt the need for it this time. 'Because we had so long between patients on the day, we all chatted about it then. Anyway, it wasn't horrific – we didn't have a lot of bad injuries. I've seen worse on any day of the week.'

One such day shortly afterwards – a Tuesday to be precise – I spent a second afternoon in Casualty. Remembering my March visit, I was anticipating a frenzy of activity, but the department was quite sedate. Janet was just about to go off duty, leaving three staff nurses on, the most senior of whom was Sister Debbie Pitt, and several students. There were just seven patients written up on the board and Janet told me, with relief, that the beds situation had been better recently. 'Usually once the new financial year comes in, in April, there's a big push to start spending money again, on surgery and bits and pieces like that. Perhaps that's been happening and they're having a better turnover on the wards. Anyway, we've only had a few overnighters this week.'

Today, only two of the seven patients were waiting for beds and Janet thought they would get them by the end of the day. According to the board, the occupied cubicles were:

CUBICLE 2: John, chest pains, waiting for a bed.
CUBICLE 4: Hannah, a young woman who'd had a termination on Friday and who had come in because she was bleeding.
CUBICLE 8: Steven, 30, with a swollen elbow.

CUBICLE 9: Molly who had dizziness and nausea. She was waiting for a bed.
CUBICLE 11: Susan, abdominal pain.
CUBICLE 13: Esther, a 72-year-old woman with a wrist injury.
CUBICLE 14: Avril, 43, with a cricked neck.

I arrived at 3.15, just as handover was taking place. One of the outgoing nurses was briefing the students and Sister Debbie on the status of the patients. It was a good-humoured occasion on the whole, as the nurses weren't too rushed, though Debbie was shocked to hear that Avril in cubicle 14 had cricked her neck last Friday. 'She's been bedbound ever since,' the outgoing nurse said, half amused, half wary, 'and she says she's been in great pain. She came in this afternoon by ambulance.'

Debbie's mouth went into an ominous line. 'A little bit of health education is in order here,' she said in the direction of cubicle 14. She then explained to the students that Avril would need a collar and painkillers, that the injury did not warrant an ambulance and that 'a person of forty-three shouldn't sit on it for five days without doing something about it!' (Debbie looked to be in her late twenties and a match for any erring patient of any age.)

After handover, the incoming nurses dispersed to the cubicles, to check on the patients. Debbie went into number 13 to see Esther. While she was in there, Esther's sister came out. She was a healthy-looking woman in her sixties or perhaps seventies, dressed in good casual clothes and wearing well-applied make-up. She asked me if I was a doctor, and when I explained what I was doing she said anxiously: 'Oh well, can you tell me, is this a *good* hospital? My sister and I are over here from America and she fell down just now when we were getting off a bus and hurt her wrist. The taxi driver just brought us straight here. We don't know anything about the hospital and I was just wondering, you know, has she been brought to a *good* place?' She trailed off and I suddenly saw the scuffed linoleum and the drab walls through her eyes.

'Very good indeed. The best,' I assured her, all at once overcome with vicarious pride. 'I know it looks run down, but the doctors and nurses here are excellent. Honestly, Alf's is famous all over the world.' She looked unconvinced, but she nodded politely. Then as Debbie emerged from cubicle 13, she went back in, perhaps reassured, perhaps not.

Twenty minutes later, Debbie caught sight of a male doctor coming out of Esther's cubicle. She hadn't seen him go in and she was annoyed; she demanded to know what he was doing with Esther. The doctor said she was having a haemotoma reduction: they'd reduce the blood swelling in the arm and put it in plaster. 'I'm fed up with no one telling me what's going on!' said Debbie. 'But you haven't been around,' protested the doctor and made for the doctor's office. Debbie was having none of it: she followed him in angrily, arguing.

Janet passed them on her way off duty; hearing Debbie's raised voice, she grinned. 'Round here she's known as Sister Debbie Pit Bull,' she murmured as she went out.

Five minutes later, after quite a bit of wrangling, Debbie emerged and explained carefully to a student what Esther was having done. She then took her off to show her what needed preparing. Debbie was aggressive but assiduous. I pressed myself against the wall, not wanting to draw any fire on to myself, but I couldn't help admiring her thoroughness. I was fairly sure that there would be no messages going astray today.

And indeed, the shift continued very smoothly. At 4 p.m. a doctor put a collar on Avril and prescribed a painkilling injection; Debbie instructed a student to get the drugs from the cupboard and then inspected then.

At 4.10, the bed manager came in to tell Debbie that a

bed had finally been found for Molly, the patient needing admission.

While they were talking, Hannah left her cubicle, looking pale, and followed a student nurse to the X-ray department.

Debbie now went in to see Avril. She was exasperated to learn that Avril's husband, who had turned up briefly, had gone off again and Avril had no idea how she was to get home. She came out shaking her head. 'I'm trying to persuade her to organize independent transport. I've told her we'll get her a taxi if there's no other option, and if her husband's at home, he can pay for it.' But Avril, it was clear, was not amenable.

A young, sporty-looking man with smart casuals and a smart accent came out of cubicle 8: it was Steven of the hurt elbow. He presented himself at the nurses' station as he'd evidently been told to, and a doctor gave him a prescription, saying that he should come back on Friday if there was no improvement. A student nurse went to wipe his name off the board. 'You're Steven, aren't you?' she said. 'Stephen with a ph actually,' he said, then added in obvious embarrassment, 'but it doesn't matter.' He walked off quickly, seeming glad to leave. He appeared uncomfortable to have been there at all and, strictly speaking, he was right to feel uncomfortable: his was one of the injuries that should really be treated by a GP.

It was now 4.30 and there was a lull. Debbie went off to one of the offices, announcing that she was going to 'sort out some triage', in other words, look through the cards of patients waiting outside and call in those most in need.

Becky, one of the staff nurses, took the opportunity to get on the telephone to a ward and follow up a little boy who had been admitted through the department yesterday. He had been seen previously at another London hospital and the A & E nurses were worried about his circumstances. They had mentioned it to the ward at the time; now Becky was checking up, asking the nurse at the other end to make sure that the boy's GP was contacted and a visit from his health visitor arranged.

It was a very different scene from that which I had left behind on my last visit. This was the pace at which A & E could run impeccably and as far as I could see, impeccably was just how it was running, patient follow up, informal health education and all. I was beginning to understand what Janet meant when she said that no two days were ever alike.

ROSTERED SERVICE began in April for the students on the adult branch. From now on they would be counted in official staff numbers and expected to take their share of the workload wherever they were placed. They would be doing regular shifts, including unsocial hours and nights, and they might be on duty for up to ten days without a break.

While on rostered service, their placements would last from five to ten weeks. They had no say in where they were sent or when. Coming up to this first placement, they had all been apprehensive and they knew it would be testing. With nice timing, it was due to end just before an important nursing exam which they would have to pass in order to stay on the course.

The students found themselves in widely differing disciplines for this first placement. Angela was on an acute surgery ward at Wavetree. Jane went on to a cardiac ward at Wavetree. Tim was on a women's ward at the Markham. Corinne went to Greville neurology ward at Alf's and Emily was on Preston, the oncology (cancer) ward.

Ever since Emily had been told of her destination, several weeks earlier, she had been in two minds. She was looking forward to getting on to a ward where she could settle in and become a real part of the team, but she was worried that she wouldn't be able to cope. According to a friend who had already worked on Preston, the nursing was specialized and many of the patients were terminal. 'That was my main worry about coming in to nursing – how was I going to cope with people dying and with other people's grief and their attempts to come to terms with it? I'm quite a weepy person and sometimes you need to be able to keep yourself in control to be any help to someone else.'

Emily's first few days on Preston did nothing to reassure her. The twenty-five-bed ward was full of patients with Hickman lines, attached to drips and bags. Many of the people looked very sick: they were pale, they had bruising from subcutaneous bleeding and some had lost their hair. Although Emily had been prepared theoretically for these symptoms (they are side effects of the chemotherapy), the sight of them was quite shocking.

Blood cancers, in which Preston specializes, are almost always treated with chemotherapy. Patients get intensive courses of powerful drugs in order to kill off the abnormal cells in the bone marrow. Because the disease destroys platelets in the blood, which help the blood to clot, patients are at risk of severe bleeding. Moreover, because the drugs destroy normal cells as well as diseased ones, their resistance to infection is low. For reasons of hygiene and comfort many people receive chemotherapy via Hickman lines.

Preston consists of several four-bedded bays and some individual side rooms. It is a mixed ward, with bays designated all male or all female. The patients on Preston were aged from eighteen to ninety. Emily learnt that they were all in different stages of disease: some of them were newly diagnosed and receiving their first course of chemotherapy while others were suffering a recurrence of the disease after having been in remission, sometimes for years. Not everyone was in for chemotherapy: some were being monitored, receiving blood transfusions or getting treatment for secondary symptoms associated with their disease.

The newly diagnosed patients were usually in side rooms,

to give them privacy and time to get used to the diagnosis. Also in side rooms were people who contracted infections and those who were going to die soon.

The nurses were welcoming and ready to help Emily. Staffing levels were good (blood cancers, especially leukaemia, attract high levels of funding and charity money): there was a senior sister, two junior sisters and a night sister. On most shifts, there would be two nurses for two patients: a qualified nurse, a student and perhaps also an oncology student (a qualified nurse doing a post-registration course). For the most part the staff knew the patients well and were ready to help Emily find her way round. The ward was bright and equipped with a kitchen and a day room, which the fitter patients were encouraged to use. Compared to other parts of Alf's, Preston was like a hotel.

None of this diluted the incredible sense of strain Emily felt during her first week there. In fact, it added to it: she felt that the staff nurses were entitled to expect more experience and knowledge from her than she could offer. Nurses were divided into three teams and each team had certain patients to look after. Because students are not allowed to handle Hickman lines, Emily wasn't involved in administering chemotherapy, but she carried out such tasks as she was permitted – the rather basic ones of taking observations, giving bed baths and mouth washes, serving food – with ferocious concentration. She went home every night with a headache and dreamed about the ward when she slept.

At the end of a week, feeling ragged, she went to see a friend who was a staff nurse on another ward, where Emily knew they had Project 2000 students. She asked for her advice on what standard of care to aim for. 'She was brilliant. She said, "Look. No one has any expectations of you. Everyone feels this way when they start a new ward. Everyone feels totally incompetent, and you still feel that way when you qualify. It's not unusual." It was an *enormous* relief.'

The following week, Emily allowed herself to ease up. She began to get to know the patients and chat to the staff. She soon found that this was almost as great a relief for them as for her: one of the junior sisters confided that they had all been wondering if there was something wrong with her because she was so intense about everything.

During her eight weeks on Preston, the range of clinical tasks Emily could do remained limited. But she got to know several of the patients very well and with them she worked at the more intangible skills involved in oncology nursing: listening to patients, supporting them through their changing reactions to their illness, helping them handle the often distressing chemotherapy.

Three weeks after Emily began on Preston, thirty-six-year-old Brian was admitted. He was very shocked to be on the ward at all: he had gone to his GP because he was finding it hard to shake off a bout of flu and thought he might need a vitamin supplement. The GP had sent him for tests and he had been diagnosed as having leukaemia. 'The next thing he knows is that he's in a ward, having a Hickman line inserted which needs to be done in the theatre; starting a course of chemotherapy; being asked to donate a sperm sample because after the chemotherapy he's likely to be infertile.'

This kind of speed is clinically necessary: the earlier chemotherapy begins, the better the chance of remission. But it is traumatic for the patient. Brian was admitted in the afternoon, his Hickman line operation scheduled for the following day. Emily was on night duty for his first, sleepless night on the ward, and she sat and talked to him for most of it.

'He wasn't on my team, but on night duty there are fewer of you and you all look after everyone. He's a Christian and I am too, and I think that made things easier in some ways. He looks at his life as being in God's hands and takes a lot of strength from that, and as a Christian I was able to talk to him about that, which means that you build up quite a good rapport. If that's someone's coping mechanism, I can understand.

'We discuss our patients in terms of how they're coping and what sort of coping mechanisms they're using and one of the nurses said about him, "Well, that's all well and good until he dies." But I think she was missing the point. To him, it was crucial and helped him cope with what was going on. His wife shares his faith too. But it doesn't stop one from feeling utterly destroyed. You know, your life's going along and you've got this idea of how it's going and then all of a sudden you're handed this.'

Brian told Emily that he was an engineer for an expanding electronics company. He had just been put in charge of a new project, which was a big break for him and amidst all his other worries he kept hoping that he wasn't going to lose his chance. The doctors had told him that if he responded well to chemotherapy and went into remission, he had a good chance of going back to work.

The next day he had his Hickman line inserted and that night Emily was on duty again. His platelets had gone very low and he started haemorrhaging from the site of the Hickman line insertion. The nurses were going every hour to check on him and give him platelets by transfusion.

The haemorrhaging stopped but Brian was weak and tired, and he was kept under observation for a few days before chemotherapy was started.

'During the chemotherapy, you're incredibly susceptible to infections. One gentleman we had recently died of septic shock, which is when you are completely overwhelmed by infection and all your major organs start to fail you. He was in his first course of chemotherapy and he was fine one minute, and the next his temperature was sky high and he died within a couple of days. But that's rare. Brian should go into first remission.'

Remission is achieved when the diseased cells are cleared from the bone marrow and bloodstream. It usually takes a few courses of chemotherapy to get a patient into remission. The first course is likely to involve their staying in hospital a few weeks; then they will return home for rest and monitoring before the next course, which will be shorter, perhaps just a few days.

During remission, which can last years, patients often return to a more or less normal life. They are regularly monitored for signs of diseased cells and when these reappear, they have more chemotherapy. If a second remission is achieved, it is usually shorter than the first. Subsequent remissions will be shorter still.

'Some people will go into remission for about ten years – Brian might. And some people will never get the disease back, but on the whole most people get it again some time in their life. Some doctors do call remission a cure: if you've got no leukaemia cells in your blood or bone marrow you are effectively cured, but that's not what you or me would call a cure. So it causes some confusion.'

Emily had her share of death on Preston. Vincent, the man who died of septic shock, was one of her patients. He was a quiet man, married with two children aged eight and twelve. He belonged to a Pentecostal Church and although he was reserved, he talked to Emily about his faith during the ten days that they were on the ward together. He became very ill one night, while she was doing her 'obs'. 'He said he was feeling unwell and he developed a very high temperature. So we told the doctor and the doctor put him on antibiotics and I kept popping in to see how he was. He was acting in a way that you would expect from someone with a high temperature, but no more than that.

'A little while later he went to the toilet and he came out without his pyjama bottoms on, which was totally out of character for him, and he seemed quite confused. We reported this. And his breathing had become very laboured and I took his observations and felt his pulse down by his wrist and it was very rapid and faint and also his blood pressure was dropping quite severely – this all happened in the course of an hour.

'The doctor came in and the sister came in; he was given drugs to try and get his blood pressure high, and all sorts of infusions to try and expand his blood volume, because in shock all the blood pools in the main organs so you risk losing the supply around the brain, and also things start to pack up. So from that point onward there was a hive of activity round his bed and I slipped away because I didn't know what was going on.'

The next day, while Emily was off duty, Vincent was transferred to intensive care. He died there a couple of days later.

Emily was not as upset as she had expected to be. 'Perhaps it was because I was expecting it. And because we share the same faith, I believe he's with God now, and I take a lot of comfort from that. And I only briefly saw his wife and his brother; I think it's other people's distress that often brings it home to you.'

She had also found it a help that, through doing observations and reporting what she found, she'd been able to take an active part in Vincent's care. She had been part of a team that had done all it could for him, even if it hadn't been able to save him in the end.

It was more difficult to do anything tangible for Derek, a man in the last stages of cancer, who had become confused. 'He'd be sitting in a chair and then suddenly he was down the ward and we effectively gave him two beds. He'd get up and say, "Where's my bed? Where's my bed?" and he'd get very agitated. I walked him up the corridor and showed him his bed, but he was extremely tired and thought he was going to collapse and I was asked to stay with him. I stayed for two hours.

'I found it very distressing because he was so distressed.

He kept on saying, "I've got to go home, I've got to see my wife." This was the morning and his wife was coming that afternoon. We'd tell him, "Your wife's coming this afternoon" and sometimes he'd seem to understand and sometimes he wouldn't. Towards the end of the two hours he was begging me to let him go home. He was saying, "Please let me go home. I'm going to die." But there was no way we could: he could hardly walk to the end of the corridor and his wife couldn't cope.'

Emily was acutely aware that these were Derek's last hours. 'It's an enormous privilege to know that you're sharing the last hours of someone's life. I've got to make these good hours. I've got to talk about things. I've got to make a difference because I'm the only one who's going to do it.'

But Derek was too ill for talking. 'There was nothing I could say and nothing I could do. Sometimes he would seem to be about to go to sleep and I would massage his hands and he would look at what I was doing.' He died that night.

Five patients died while Emily was on Preston. It sounds a lot, but as she pointed out, it represented a small percentage of the patients she cared for during two months on a twenty-five bed ward, especially as some beds were occupied by a series of short-stay patients.

'There was one lady I looked after – I think she had leukaemia – she got a condition which is extremely painful and makes it hard to drink or swallow. She was in on infusion to keep her hydrated but she's gone home now. Then there was another lady who kept on getting nosebleeds because her platelets were getting very low – she comes in for a day or so every two or three days, then goes home again.

'And these are the people who are actually ill. That's the problem with being in hospital – you don't see the people who've had leukaemia for five years but are leading relatively normal lives.'

These people are catered for by a weekly clinic, held at

Alf's. The staff nurses on Preston were encouraging Emily to visit it. There, they told her, she would see people who had formerly been in-patients on Preston, who now went to the clinic just once a month for a check over and a chat. 'These people are perfectly well, have been perfectly well for five or six years, and have almost forgotten that they had leukaemia or lymphoma.'

Emily intended to go to the clinic when she could find the time. But time was a problem. There was a vast amount to learn about nursing cancer patients. (For instance, chemotherapy is a subject in itself, with its side effects of mouth sores, nausea, hair loss and fatigue, the ways in which patients react to such symptoms and the ways in which nursing and medicine can alleviate them.) Emily knew much more now than when she had started on Preston, but she also knew that her knowledge was 'a drop in the ocean'.

ON GREVILLE neurology ward, Corinne was finding the work unexpectedly interesting. It was a thirty-two-bed ward for patients with brain disorders and it was surgically orientated: patients were either preparing for or recovering from operations. Many patients had brain tumours or aneurysms (a sac formed by abnormal dilation of the weakened wall of a blood vessel); some had fluid on the brain, which needed to be drained; others had varying degrees of brain damage after road traffic accidents. There were also rarer disorders, like having no resistance to pain. And the ward treated certain spinal problems as well.

The Project 2000 course had barely touched on this area of medicine, so to prepare herself Corinne read through some booklets. She started the placement feeling that it was all completely new to her.

One of the first things that struck her was the pace of the work. The heart of Greville is an eight-bed recovery ward, where patients come immediately after theatre. During the first hours after the operation, nurses have to take observations every fifteen minutes, which involve checking patients' eyes for response to stimuli, checking their limbs for movements and taking pulse and blood pressure readings. In some cases – if a patient is diabetic, for instance – the nurse will have to do a pin-prick blood test every so often. As patients come round (usually within a few hours), the time between observations is lengthened, but they remain very regular while the patient recovers strength and faculties. This recovery depends on all kinds of factors: the patient's age and fitness; the success of the operation; the nature of the disorder. Some patients recover well within days; others take weeks, or longer.

Once patients are less dependent, they are moved into one of the four- or six-bed bays to regain strength and be monitored.

Because the work is demanding, staffing levels are fairly high. The ward had a senior sister and two junior sisters, and in total eight nurses were supposed to be on each shift. Agency nurses were used regularly to make up numbers.

Corinne found the staff approachable and friendly, and the sister gave her time to settle in. She was assigned a mentor: Judy was a staff nurse of twenty-six who had only just started on the ward herself, after completing a post-registration neurology course. Corinne liked her but could have done with someone more experienced to show her the ropes. 'She treats me as a colleague rather than a student. She's not very motivated to teach: she'll grumble about her shifts being switched and she'll confide in me. She says she still needs to find her feet herself.'

For the first couple of weeks, Corinne chose to do most things with Judy. 'The patients were so dependent, I felt I wanted to be supervised.' She did observations which she found 'a handful. You've got to be always on guard. For instance, all the patients are on anti-convulsant tablets because any disorder of the brain can cause a fit. So you have to monitor them very closely and be aware of what a fit looks like: it can be just a twitch of the face.'

She was picking up information from the staff nurses as she went. Some of it came by observation, some of it by semi-formal instruction: one of the junior sisters had sat down with her early on and explained the structure of the brain and the main problems seen on Greville. In addition, the ward held classes once a week for all the students, Project 2000 and RGN, to teach them the essentials of neurology. Corinne found these very useful: 'Once you understand what can go wrong with the brain, you can be more prepared to care for patients.'

She also went down to theatre to see a brain operation being performed. 'It was on a man who had no resistance to pain. He had stimulants – wires – put into the first layer of his brain, going down into his chest, where there's a little computerized monitor pre-set to control the pain.' (The wires run in the fatty layer beneath the skin. The procedure has similarities with the shunt operation Rachel witnessed.)

'There's another man on the ward who had this done but his wires got infected so they had to be taken out. He's on antibiotics now, and waiting to have the same operation again. He's not very optimistic, because he says that the wires didn't control his pain anyway. But the second man, whose operation I saw, it worked for him very well. He went home after seven days.'

After three weeks, Corinne was given two patients to look after. 'There's one who basically just needs tender, loving care. She's a seventy-eight year-old; she had a subarachnoid haemorrhage – it's a tumour-type thing, so they operated on it but they don't really think she's going to pull through. It was a week ago now and she's not conscious. Her family's been informed, so basically we're just doing the activities of daily living for her – cleaning her, washing her, spending time with her. She's on morphine.'

The other patient was Liam, twenty-one, who had been in a road accident with his wife: a taxi had run into them. His wife hadn't been badly hurt but Liam had a brain haemorrhage and was brought in unconscious. The surgeons put leads into his brain; they would remain there in the short term to drain the blood away as it continued to pool. For days Liam remained unconscious and Corinne and the other nurses carried out fifteen-minute observations and tried to stimulate him. 'Basically it's observations on his eyes and for power in his arms – seeing if he's got movement back in his limbs.'

Liam was in a semi-coma. He could be moved into a sitting position, and staff were encouraged to walk around him and talk to him, trying to get a response. Two days went by and there was nothing, until on the afternoon of the third day, Corinne and one of the junior sisters were standing by his bed, doing his observations. 'He was just sitting there in a daze like he normally is and suddenly he spoke, out of the blue. The sister, she just burst out crying she was so pleased!'

Corinne looked shy when I asked what her own feelings had been, and agreed, 'it was great'. Voluble about practical things, she did not easily put her emotions into words.

As the eight weeks went on, Corinne took on more responsibility. She took thirty stitches out of a patient's head ('it pained me more than him') and was given a new patient to look after: Kay, a twenty-eight-year-old who came in with headaches and dizziness and whose X-ray showed an aneurysm. 'That's when two arteries grow into each other and blood accumulates. It can be fatal if it bursts, so she had an operation the next day, where the arteries are clipped. It's what the majority of our patients come in with; 2 per cent of the population have it.'

Kay also had a temporary drain put in, to draw off excess

blood. The operation was successful and she recovered quite fast. A constant stream of relatives and friends visited her, and Corinne got to know some of them quite well. 'It's part of what I'm learning here. It's one of the things I like about rostered service – I'm learning how to approach patients' families and treat patients as a whole rather than just an illness. Non-verbal communication is important on this ward too, because some of the patients can't speak – you learn to read their facial expressions and to ask them how they are.'

In the last week of the placement, I went on the ward with Corinne. It was a hot afternoon and the sun shone relentlessly through the large windows into the recovery ward. It seemed very quiet: at first I thought only half the beds were full, but a closer look showed that those which seemed empty were occupied by sleeping or semi-conscious patients. In fact, seven of the eight beds were filled and the other was awaiting a patient due up from surgery. The bed itself was missing, having been wheeled down to the theatre; next to its space a 'Nil By Mouth' notice was Sellotaped to the Anglepoise lamp in preparation.

Corinne gave me a quick resumé of the patients: down one side of the ward lay a young Chinese woman who'd had an hydrocephalus drain put in; an elderly woman who'd had an aneurysm operated on four weeks ago and whose recovery had been delayed by complications; and a man with facial cancer who'd just had a massive operation to remove the diseased tissue.

On the other side a middle-aged woman was sitting up and talking to her husband; she'd been in a week awaiting an operation due five days ago and cancelled. She was often confused and dysphasic (forgetting the correct words for things), although at the moment she sounded very lucid. There was a woman in her thirties with a newly shaved patch on her head; she had gone down to the theatre that morning but the oxygen equipment had been faulty and the operation had been postponed. 'She and her mother are furious. That's her mother sitting with her now; we're hoping she won't sue.' Another woman was sitting in a wheelchair, with a bandaged head, a nasogastric tube in and a monitor attached to her: she'd had her operation ten days before. And there was Kay, asleep at the moment and well on the mend.

'I took her drain out yesterday, unsupervised,' Corinne said. 'You have to take stitches out of a large cut on the head and draw the tube out slowly. She was in a lot of pain and I thought I must be doing something wrong, but when I got the staff nurse to come and supervise me, she said it was fine.'

There was no bustle on the ward. The staff did observations without fuss and often without disturbing the sleeping patients. The results were written up diligently in the notes: Corinne showed me one of the patients' observation charts spanning several days and the amount of information recorded was extraordinary – it included not only medically quantifiable things like pulse rate and pupil reactions, but requests the patient had made for food and the nurses' impressions of the patient's moods and well-being.

For quite a while that afternoon it was hard for me to get a sense of exactly what the nurses were doing. It was only when a mishap was averted, such as when the woman in the wheelchair tried to move suddenly, and nearly pulled her monitor down on top of her, or when discomfort was allayed – the semi-conscious elderly woman moaned and Corinne closed her curtains to protect her from the heat of the sun – that I realized what Corinne meant by having to be on your guard. Many of these patients were so helpless that the nurses had to be their eyes and their hands.

When I asked Corinne if it was normally this quiet, she said that it would change when the patient returned from surgery. Then, for an hour or so, the activity round her would be intensive.

It was a Monday and Corinne's last day on the ward before

she had to sit the big nursing exam on Thursday. She was going to spend the next two days studying hard, as the pressure of adapting to rostered service, together with the need to learn about neurology on the job, had made it difficult for her to revise. After the exam, she would come straight back on to Greville for her last three shifts here, working Friday, Saturday and Sunday. And then, I asked, a break? No, then she would go straight to her next placement: this time next week she would be beginning ten weeks in cardiology.

WHILE THE adult branch students found themselves catapulted into the heart of ward work, Nicola's spring placement took her a step away from the hospital. She was to spend a month with a community psychiatric nurse, visiting patients in their homes.

Community Psychiatric Nurses (CPNs) are a growing breed, vitally important for the operation of care in the community. CPNs visit people who are suffering from mental illness or severe emotional problems; they give counselling, supervise any medication the patients take and monitor their condition. In an ideal world, or even one which delivered on its promises, there would be enough CPNs to go round.

Over the last few years, residential homes and hospitals for the mentally ill have been closing down. Wavetree had a fairly large number of these, and so has discharged many people with mental health problems into the community. Recognizing the need for CPNs, it employs quite a few – not enough, but as many as its budget can stretch to.

At first, Nicola was optimistic about the placement. She was assigned to a CPN named Miriam, who had already supervised one of her friends on the course. Nicola had heard encouraging things about Miriam and, when they met, she was impressed by the fact that Miriam was well versed in the Project 2000 approach.

'She had a student folder and had read through the objectives I had to do and made out a plan with me to achieve them, which was basically doing assessments and planning care, looking after people in their own homes and dealing with how different that is from being in institutions.'

CPNs work in teams: each area has a team, which works in conjunction with local hospitals, general practices and health centres to identify people in need of CPN care. Each individual CPN then has her (or his) own geographical patch to cover, and visiting is done one on one, with the CPN seeing clients in their homes.

Miriam's patch was in west Wavetree, encompassing a large, poor council estate. Her clients were adults spanning the age range from eighteen to sixty-five. (Once people are over sixty-five, their care is provided by 'care of the elderly' teams.) Nicola's four weeks were spent visiting the various clients at weekly intervals and doing a certain amount of liaison work with hospitals and GPs.

She soon realized that much of her time would be spent observing Miriam. There were no simple physical tasks a student could help with and their visits were time-limited and structured around conversations between Miriam and the clients. During them, Nicola would usually just sit quietly, watch and listen; afterwards, she and Miriam would talk things over.

The clients had a diversity of problems. There was Richard, in his fifties, who had been on medication for depression, and whose wife and children had left him. After they left he had stopped taking his medication and his mental state had worsened: he'd begun to think his neighbours were watching him and stealing from him (fears and paranoia about neighbours are quite common in mental illness), and he also believed his wife was watching him to see if he was with another woman. He'd been admitted to hospital after smashing his neighbours' door down, and once he'd recovered enough to be discharged, Miriam was assigned to him.

She and Nicola went to see him in Wilcox Ward at Alf's shortly before the discharge. They introduced themselves and agreed a date to visit him at home; on that visit Nicola made the formal assessment. 'It was the first one I'd done, though I'd sat and listened to Miriam doing them before. In the assessment you're finding out about his personal situation, what he believes brought him into hospital, what sort of situation he's in now, what sort of support he's got, what are the likely problems, how much support is he going to need from you. You work from quite a detailed questionnaire, but you don't sit there writing it up – that would look very officious – you use it as a guideline and fill it in afterwards. You have to be careful how you do it because some people might think you were checking up on them, but he was fine about it. I think he was glad to be home and realized he needed some support. And Miriam has a very nice manner; she's able to be a nurse to people and at the same time a friend.'

There is very little hands-on physical care in a CPN's job. A high proportion of the work – Nicola estimated about 60–70 per cent – is counselling. Miriam had done a counselling course and employed a mixture of behavioural and cognitive techniques. Behaviour therapy means helping the client manage their symptoms of fear and distress, usually by giving them physical or mental exercises to practise. A cognitive approach looks at the thoughts and emotions which lead to the behaviour.

'To me the cognitive approach makes more sense. The behavioural approach is more like treating people as animals who are just acting on instinct – irrational behaviour. But I believe there is always an underlying reason. I like to know what's behind this behaviour, not just get rid of it, because it can just develop into something else. A mixture of cognitive and behavioural work is good.'

Miriam was adopting this kind of mixture with Kemal who had been referred to her by his GP. Kemal was a retired widower who had begun suffering from panic attacks so severe he was almost blacking out. 'The panic attacks make him feel he's choking. He feels the air is only getting so far, he'll be breathing very quickly and then getting light-headed because he's taking in too much oxygen. There is a very physiological basis to the sensation and once Miriam explained it to him and he understood it, he was much calmer. It also helped him to know he wasn't the only one to have panic attacks. Miriam taught him deep breathing exercises to do, not only when he's feeling panicky but at various times. And she's got him started on anti-depressants. He was sleeping badly, not eating, classic symptoms of depression.'

As well as offering Kemal these very practical forms of help, Miriam talked to him at length and elicited some of the background to his stress, helping him recognize what had driven him to this point. 'He's got two grown-up children and he's someone who has always been there for other people. He had a friend who had a breakdown and he watched him getting worse and worse and was terrified that was going to happen to him. I think perhaps he couldn't take any more and this was a way of withdrawing. He is getting better as the weeks go by.'

As the weeks went by, too, Nicola was building her impressions of community psychiatric nursing. On the one hand, she liked what she saw of Miriam's counselling skills and felt that she was gaining an insight into how they worked. This was important, as her lectures had covered only the basic precepts of counselling, looking at a few of the counselling models in use and doing some role playing. Now she could study the real thing.

'A lot of it is showing that you are listening; if someone makes a throw-away remark, it's picking it up. It's not telling people what they should be doing, it's helping people work it out for themselves. Though some people do need a more directive approach – then you try and do it subtly. What I like about going into people's homes is it's very much their territory. In hospitals it's very easy to fall into being bossy. I do try not to do it but I see it around me, whereas in someone's house, you're there as a guest. It makes it more equal.'

On the other hand, she was angered by the gap that existed between the rhetoric and the reality of community care. Going on rounds with Miriam, she could see clearly how the CPNs struggled to deal with a rising tide of demand, and how poor living conditions contributed to people's problems in the first place then impeded their recovery. It also became plain that the closure of the institutions (which she welcomed) had not been replaced with the promised network of support services.

'There's a move within community psychiatric nursing to take nurses away from what is disparagingly termed "the worried well" – these are people who don't cause society a lot of problems: they're quietly unhappy, people with phobias, depression and anxiety – and resources are going to be concentrated on the visibly ill or visibly mentally distressed. Schizophrenics for instance, who actually make a noise and are visible and perhaps cause damage. I think CPNs are going to find themselves dealing more and more with these people. That's certainly what's going to happen in Wavetree because resources are so stretched that people who aren't literally falling apart at the seams are just going to have to cope.'

She was angry at what she saw as the cynical government approach. She had believed in the principles of care in the community, she still did. But it had taken only a few weeks out in that community to see that those principles were far from being enacted. In fact, she was inclined to think the government's fine words were only a smokescreen. 'Community care is being implemented with no extra money. It has been brought in to look like an altruistic thing you're doing for people's benefit, but really it's a cost-cutting exercise. Psychiatric hospitals are too expensive to run, so they're shutting them down and developing the buildings and the land. What's more they are taking health out of the notion of community care; they are putting social workers in charge of organising it,* health is taking a back seat and we are going to be focusing on social control.'

Nicola seemed to have become disillusioned in an alarmingly short space of time. It was not all down to the CPN placement, though: she said that doubts and disappointments had been accumulating gradually for months and in the last few weeks they had reached critical mass. She was especially worried by the creeping element of social control in psychiatric nursing. In theory, for instance, the CPN's job was the least authoritarian nursing role she had come across. But this was under threat: the government was proposing to introduce Community Supervision Orders, whereby patients who were living in their own homes could be compelled to receive supervision and medication from the CPNs. As clients frequently stop taking medication or ask to change it (usually because they can't stand the side effects) this would radically alter the relationship between CPNs and their clients, turning CPN's into warders and clients into legal charges. It's a far cry from the idea of the nurse as the patient's advocate.

As it stands, it is part of the CPN's job to administer drugs where prescribed and where clients are willing to take them. CPNs need to be aware of the possible side effects (which can be significant, such as stiffness, uncontrollable twitching or all round slowing down); to monitor the clients carefully and be ready to adjust the dose or change the drug. This is

* There is a financial/political angle to this: care which is devolved to social services is paid for out of local authority money, rather than funded directly by central government. Officially, therefore, the government is no longer the provider of such services and can distance itself from any cuts. In some cases, too, people may lose their statutory right to services which switch from 'health' to 'social'. These can then be cut without fear of legal liability.

done by reporting back to the doctor (either GP or hospital doctor) and making recommendations. Miriam told Nicola that very often she would tell the GP what to prescribe and the dose, and they would do it without question. In some cases this was due to the GP's lack of interest; in others, an awareness that Miriam knew the clients better than they did.

The whole question of medication within psychiatry is a vexed one, and Nicola was feeling her way around it cautiously. 'The range of medication is getting bigger and there are some drugs now with fewer side effects. But they all have some drawbacks. Some of them work very well in suppressing voices and visions, so people put up with the side effects. Sometimes they would rather have the hallucinations. I don't think they should be forced to take medication.

'One of my questions is whether they will ever be free of it, once they're on it. Good GPs and psychiatrists review it regularly and try to cut down as much as possible; they'll give the patient drug-free periods to see what happens. I think generally it's a long-term thing and that's where the danger is – in cumulative, irreversible side effects – which is tragic.'

Of course, prescribing medication depends on diagnosis, which is an equally complex issue. Nicola was very reluctant to approach patients in terms of diagnosis; indeed, she thought it dangerous. The more she went on rounds with Miriam, the more she believed that living conditions, education and social confidence (or lack of it) were hugely important factors in the way society defined 'mental illness'.

For instance, one of Miriam's clients was a woman who lived in a two-bedroomed flat with her five sons, aged seven to fifteen. The flat was cramped and in a high-rise block; she and her sons were half Bengali and half English and suffering racial intimidation from neighbours. Since she had been attacked on the walkways she wouldn't leave the flat and kept her sons away from school in turns to keep her company.

Miriam was campaigning on her behalf with the council,

trying to get her moved, without much success. Meanwhile she visited the woman to give her support and someone to talk to. Which was all very well, but as Nicola said, who wouldn't be depressed and at the end of their tether in such circumstances?

The diagnosis-led approach, Nicola believed, ignored these human truths. The day before I met her, Nicola had sat in the local health centre with a psychiatrist who was reviewing progress in some of Miriam's clients. 'This guy came in and he seemed fine to me, a little quiet but he was answering her questions. When he went out she turned to me and said, "Chronic schizophrenic, latent affect," and reeled off these symptoms. I thought, did I miss something?

'But she was looking at him in that narrow view psychiatrists often take – they want the patient to fit with their diagnosis. I'd been watching her and she would say to him what she wanted to hear. She'd say: "So you're feeling such and such, am I right?" And then afterwards she said to me, "He didn't say much!" '

The placement drew to a close and Nicola now concentrated on preparing for the exam which loomed ahead at the end of June. The mental health branch exam was different from the adult branch, but students sat them in the same week. She had revision to do, and a project to finish, which would count towards her final mark: the subject was a journal of her work with one patient. She had chosen Mrs Green, from Morris Ward, and now that she was completing the paper, she looked in on the ward to see how her favourite was doing. She found her with her bags packed, imperiously waiting for a taxi she had called.

'She'd discharged herself. They weren't really doing anything to find out what was behind the handwashing and she didn't want to be there any more. Apparently she'd just called a friend and said, "I'm coming!" I went down to the taxi with her and said, "Are you sure you'll be all right? Do you know where you're going? Have you got enough money for the taxi?" Then she was off. I don't know what'll happen to her.'

She suspected that Mrs Green would fall through the net of support services; the mesh was not in very good repair, after all.

RACHEL, MEANWHILE, had spent June doing the A & E placement which she had been dreading, at a district hospital a few miles away. Had it turned out to be a pleasant surprise?

'No, it was horrible. There were three of us that went to this particular hospital and we were totally lost. I didn't know anything, I couldn't do anything. The staff were nice but they didn't know what level we were at – they haven't even started Project 2000 there – and they didn't even know we were there for children.'

There were some good days, like the one Rachel spent with a paramedic, out on call in a car, but she spent most of her time talking to patients, doing some simple dressings and following the staff around. She had little trouble deciding that A & E was not for her: she missed the continuity of ward work and couldn't get used to the way that patients left the department for the wards and were never heard of again.

Nor did she like the way she saw some young patients being treated: 'They had some who came in for overdoses, but it was so mechanical the way they were treated and I think it was wrong. You almost felt like the staff were punishing them: "It's a horrible job, putting a tube down and pumping your stomach, and I really resent this because I don't want to do this and I don't enjoy this, and why were you so stupid?" I don't know, perhaps you do become harder if you do that every day.'

The experience had not dampened her enthusiasm for

nursing, though: it simply confirmed her suspicions that she wanted nothing to do with A & E. She looked forward to her next two placements, which would be rostered service ones, lasting ten weeks each, on Howard and Walsh. At this stage, she didn't know which would come first: she rather hoped it was Howard, as she had enjoyed it so much before.

But first, like all the other students, she had to knuckle down to revise for the June exam.

IN ST WENCESLAS, on Hamilton, life continued in its gentle rhythm. Christine's two new patients had been there long enough to start establishing a routine. Edie was fairly independent and able to articulate her likes and dislikes. She was able to choose her own clothes, request her choice of food and with help she could go to the lavatory and have baths. She had Parkinson's Disease, which made her very shaky; the nurses had to be on hand to help her with her activities and had constantly to check that she couldn't fall, or knock things over and hurt herself.

Grace was a very quiet, unassuming lady. At first Christine had found it hard to get her to express any preferences at all: 'If you asked her when she wanted her breakfast she'd say, "Any time *you* want me to have my breakfast." I'd say, "No, it's not what I want, it's what *you* want." ' But now Grace had come out of herself a little: she was able to choose her own breakfast and make decisions about when to get up and go back to bed. She had recently told Christine that her favourite colour was blue.

Grace could do many practical things for herself. She was temporarily unable to walk as she was recovering from a fractured femur, but she could stand up with help from another person and could transfer herself from one chair to another. She could wash her face, hands and the top part of her body. She could dress herself, apart from her knickers and her stockings. She could feed herself. She could stay continent during the day if she was taken regularly to the lavatory.

Christine was trying to draw Grace out of herself and engage her mentally. This had also been difficult at first, because Grace had been reluctant to let Christine sit and talk to her – she was afraid she would be wasting Christine's time. During the last two months, however, Christine had taken her out in a wheelchair to visit another ward and was now having regular 'orientation' sessions with her, during which she would use objects like photographs and plastic fruit to start conversations and draw out Grace's memories.

In June, I got the chance to meet Edie and Grace myself. After securing the permission of the department (Christine had been very anxious that the visit should be cleared), I was able to go on to Hamilton for a visit.

On 14 June, at a quarter past nine in the morning, the day room was light, almost bright with sun. Much of the rest of the ward was dim, however, with curtains still drawn around beds as the staff helped patients to dress and have their breakfasts. Most patients have breakfast either in bed or in their chairs beside it.

A few women were sitting in armchairs, around the edges of the day room. They were not talking to each other, though some were speaking in low voices to themselves. Most of them were very thin and frail and it was quite hard to put an age to them: the abstracted look on their faces seemed to set them at one remove from the ageing process.

In the middle of the room several tables were pushed together and two vases of spring flowers and a fading arrangement of irises and pinks stood on them. A white laminated noticeboard was stuck to the wall; on it purple handwriting announced 'Friday 14th June, Season: Spring, Weather: Cloudy'.

Christine was busy with her patients. She introduced me briefly to the other staff: there was Jennifer, who was giving porridge to Hilary, a diabetic lady in a curtained bed; Suzanne who was on the telephone; Renee who was here and there, being busy. At the far end of the ward was Lucy, a young girl on a youth training scheme to become a nursing assistant. A college student called Priscilla, who was doing two weeks' work experience on Hamilton, was in a half-opened cubicle with Edie.

Christine paused by the curtain and introduced me to Priscilla and Edie. Edie was dressed and sitting in her chair. She looked bewildered at the sight of me and, when Christine asked if she would like to talk to me, said, with a touch of panic, 'No. I don't want to be tired.'

There were other nurses and assistants on the ward, but it was difficult to keep track of who was who. Everyone was fully occupied and I didn't like to take up their time. Almost all the members of staff on the ward were African Caribbean, a noticeable contrast to the wards in Alf's, where the nurses were almost all white. I remembered that some of the students had remarked that, judging by their placements, African Caribbean nurses tend to be better represented in elderly care than elsewhere. Some of this may reflect a different attitude amongst African Caribbean nurses and a greater readiness to work with the elderly; much of it is undoubtedly due to the fact that elderly care employs a high proportion of enrolled nurses and auxiliaries, many of whom, for a variety of social, educational and financial reasons, are black. All but one of the patients on Hamilton were white, and I asked Christine if this caused problems: there is, after all, a fair amount of racial fear and intolerance among elderly white Londoners. Sitting in the staff room eating her cornflakes (she took breakfast at 9.45), she said it hardly ever arose; whatever they might have felt before they came into hospital, the patients showed scarcely any awareness of race once they were here. It was one of the things that simply ceased to matter.

At 10 o'clock there were nine women in the day room.

Priscilla, the college student, was helping one of them to eat breakfast. Her name was Olive and she was very thin, with a pale face and limbs that looked brittle. Next to her sat a much more robust woman: this was Susan, the most outgoing patient on the ward. She was dressed merrily in a green floral dress, a yellow cardigan, thick tan stockings and heavy boots, and her white hair was brushed flat to her head and arranged sweetly in two tiny plaits, tied with ribbon at the back. She was chatting to Olive and encouraging her to drink her tea. 'Nice cup of tea you've got there!' she kept saying in a kindly, booming voice.

One of the nurses called Priscilla away, to help her move a lady in a blue dress. It was time for this patient's exercise. Priscilla and the nurse took an arm each and manoeuvred her out of her chair; then, murmuring encouragement, they walked her a few shuffling steps to the table and back to her chair again. They settled her down with a cup of tea.

Olive was calling for Priscilla now, in a high thin voice. Susan added hers to it, eager to do something constructive, and Priscilla returned to see what was needed. Christine appeared with a cup of tea; she took it to a woman sitting silently in a pink dressing gown, a few feet from Olive and Susan. I learnt afterwards that this was Mary, who had been admitted quite recently and was another of Christine's special patients.

Mary tried to drink the tea too fast and Christine intervened with: 'No! You'll burn yourself! Drink it slowly!' Mary was deaf, and Christine repeated the message several times, her voice so loud that it was distorted, almost a shout.

Susan was now trying to have a conversation with Olive. She was asking about her family, drawing her out sympathetically, with a certain amount of expertise. I wondered how many times during the day she tried to get through to her fellow patients like this.

'I've got two daughters, that's all,' Olive said.

'How many grandchildren have you got?' chipped in Christine.

'I live in a tall building and it costs a lot of money to get a person up there,' said Olive. Then, looking straight ahead of her, her face and voice full of anguish, she went on: 'And they still won't let me die. I'm dead. I'm laid out in the cemetery.'

'You're not dead, Olive,' said Christine. 'You're here with us.'

'I want to look after her,' said Olive. 'I want to take care of her in the cemetery and make it nice. I live in my daughter's home now.' She paused and added in a desolate voice: 'They tell me I'm getting better.'

'Yes, you are,' said Priscilla. 'You talk to me every day and you're getting better all the time. You can lift your hand up now.'

'All I want to do is go to bed and stay there and sleep,' Olive told Susan. 'I don't want to know anything else.'

'Well, I don't very much either,' said Susan in a companionable tone.

Christine went away and Olive fell silent for a while. Susan began filling in with a running commentary, which seemed to be aimed at comforting Olive. 'I'm sitting back in my chair now,' she said. And, 'I'm sitting here with you. I'm chatting.'

'I've been like it a long, long time,' said Olive eventually.

'We've all got something wrong with us,' said Susan. 'Then with some of us we get better again.'

Christine reappeared and told Mary that it was time for her bath. Priscilla helped her wheel the patient away; as they went, Mary said she didn't want a bath and Christine answered her in a shout, her raised voice sounding at odds with her words, intended to comfort: 'That's all right, we'll just wash you then.'

Olive, meanwhile, had become trapped in a reminiscence about someone who went through the wars. On and on her voice went, high and sepulchral; it was expressive of an unbearable pain. Susan, in what seemed like an attempt to soothe her, said, 'I'm going to the toilet now.' All along, I realized, their conversation had been conducted in these two unrelating modes, with Susan speaking only of immediate actions and surroundings and Olive speaking only out of her memories. However, as Susan got up and walked heavily off to the lavatory, Olive looked after her and said sweetly: 'Be careful.' Then she returned to her monologue about the war, speaking into the air.

With Susan gone, I became uneasy in the day room. The women sitting around the edge of it were all locked in their own worlds, or else didn't want to talk, and the voyeurism of my position was brought home to me. I felt ashamed and went into the small office, which looked into the day room through a glass panel. There I settled down to read a catalogue of therapeutic videos, objects and games, all designed for care of the elderly. Christine had told me that she had been given permission to start a reminiscence therapy group and she was sending away for some aids in the catalogue. The ward had only a limited budget and many of the things were beyond its reach; she'd had to choose carefully.

She had marked a set of videos called *The War Years* (£40), a reminiscence quiz book 1930–1969 (£25), a *Picture Post* album 1938–1957 (£13) and 'Famous Faces' 1920–60, a set of forty cards with pictures and brief biographies of famous people. Looking through the pages at the photographs of the merchandise and the posed scenes of people using them, I saw that all the models were fit, healthy people in their sixties.

After twenty minutes, Susan came in and sat down. I anticipated a cheerful enquiry about what I was doing, but instead she grasped her breasts and said they were drooping and uncomfortable and could I do something about them? At a loss, I sympathized. Then she said that she wanted to go and see her mother but no one would take her. She began to cry. She couldn't remember which door her mother lived at.

'So many times I've just walked by the end of the street. Just gone past the door. I don't know. I don't think she'd recognize me now. She's getting on, she doesn't know who I am. She might think I'm dead and that's what worries me. She probably wouldn't even know me.'

Susan was weeping heartbrokenly. I tried to remember what Christine had said about validation therapy: 'One or two will be upset and will want to go home "to their mum". Most of them talk about their mum, as if they're going back in time. We can't tell them, "That's wrong"; that's the time to do validation therapy with them. With some of them you can say, "I think your mother died" and they will think and then say, "Yes, that's right." With others they still can't remember. Some will cry – that's a normal human reaction when you hear that someone's dead, so we let them cry.'

I could not tell this weeping woman that her mother was dead. Instead I tried to lead her on to happier memories, but she just said she couldn't talk to people any more because no one would believe her; why wouldn't anyone take her to her mother's house? She had asked and asked, but no one would take her and in any case, she didn't know if her mother would recognize her . . .

For about ten minutes she grieved and then she said humbly that she knew she was a silly bugger, this was soppy talk. Could we go and do something else? I said I was busy reading, and asked if she'd like me to take her back into the day room. Immediately she recoiled, said, 'Oh, you're busy, I'll leave you,' and struggled out of the chair. Ashamed of myself, I offered her my arm and tried to talk to her again, but she had been rebuffed: she hesitated in the doorway then went away to find Priscilla. I heard her asking Priscilla if there was anything she could do about her breasts. 'Are you wearing a bra?' Priscilla asked and, finding that she wasn't, took Susan off to find one and make her comfortable. It hadn't occurred to me to ask a simple, practical question like that.

Christine had been busy with Grace for the last forty-five minutes, helping her get up and dressed. Now she walked slowly past the office with Grace on her arm and settled her in a chair just inside the day room. She called me over to talk to her.

Grace had white hair and a composed face, with wide-spaced eyes. She spoke very quietly and lucidly, with a 'so be it' humorous turn to her words. She was evidently very weak and I had to sit close to her for her to hear me. She talked to me quite freely; I had the impression that she was trying to please me for Christine's sake.

She had been married, she told me, to a man she met 'over ten years ago'. She had been living in a home at the time, and the residents had gone on holiday to Clacton. He was there with another party, and she had struck up a friendship with him when she was seated at his table. They had married after a couple of months and moved into his family home. Grace said that she had thought his brother and sister unkind to him: they didn't even give him new underclothes, but she gave him 'the best of my attention' for two years. She repeated this several times, adding that she always gave him the best of everything, until he died. The mention of this made her cry.

We talked about further back in the past then: she had grown up in the north and worked in a mill. She laughed about how she had walked to work in clogs and a shawl. I assumed that she had been single until the meeting in Clacton but suddenly, out of a pause in the talk, she volunteered: 'I had a boy and a girl, but they didn't live very long.' She thought and then said sadly: 'It might have been better that way. If they'd lived they might have got the cancer like my husband.' She began to tell me about her husband going into hospital and how the doctor had written to say he had cancer all through him. She cried again and said that she didn't talk about him often, it was too upsetting. I said something platitudinous about memories being both happy and sad, and sometimes you needed to have the sadness to get to the good ones. I knew I was being presumptuous: these women were caught in a loop of loss and pain beyond anything I had experienced.

I remembered that Christine had mentioned a recent outing she had been on, with Grace and some of the other patients. They had gone to the nearest large park. I asked Grace if she went out at all; only when she felt like it, she said quietly, and her expression implied that this wasn't often.

I was afraid of tiring her and afraid of upsetting her, so I sat on with her in silence for a while. She looked around at the other women: a few yards away one woman sat hunched in her chair, shouting wordlessly. 'She does that most of the time,' said Grace. Then with a flash of humour she cocked her head at the woman beyond her. 'She slept most of yesterday with her slippers on the wrong feet,' she said, and laughed.

It was shortly before twelve and the lunch trolley had arrived. The nurses were beginning to organize plates and cutlery. Some patients were being walked to the table; most were having small tables put in front of them. Visitors were beginning to arrive. I shook hands with Grace and thanked her for talking to me, then I went to have a few words with Christine.

She was keen to know what Grace had said to me. She was fond of her and had started working steadily with her in informal reminiscence sessions. It surprised her that Grace had told me about her husband, as she was usually slow to talk about her personal life. And she was astonished to hear about the daughter and son: Grace had spoken of a young husband but never mentioned children. Perhaps, Christine suggested, looking at my large belly, it was because I was very noticeably pregnant myself.

She also told me that when Susan had talked about her mother, she meant her daughter, who came to visit her two or three times a week. She habitually got them confused. I was taken aback: Susan's longing had seemed so very much that of a daughter for her lost mother, a needful love, shot through with guilt and hope. But then, on reflection, that could describe an elderly mother's yearning for her daughter too. It came home to me how delicate was the process of nursing these women: a matter of listening and slow learning, disentangling the threads of language and emotion to reach a common understanding of the truth.

In many ways, nurses like Christine are the keepers of their patients' stories.

They are also their carers and helpers in the most concrete sense of the words. As I left at a quarter past twelve, some of the staff were passing plates and glasses to their patients; others were cutting up their food and helping them to eat; others were greeting the visitors – middle-aged sons and daughters, mainly – and taking them to their mothers. Christine was wheeling Mary out of the day room again. Since her bowl of cornflakes at a quarter to ten, she had not once sat down.

Summer

THE STUDENTS' EXAMS came round, as exams do. Nicola found her paper reasonable, and Rachel was delighted and relieved to discover that her tactical approach to revising – concentrate on certain subjects and hope to God they come up – had paid off. The adult branch students were less happy. The questions on their paper required very full answers and the students would have to reach a pass mark on each question in order to pass the paper as a whole.

Jane read through the questions, realized she could not answer them and left the examination room early. She had that slightly disorienting lightness of heart that comes with taking drastic action: she went shopping for the next few hours and then made her way to the pub, to meet the others and get their reactions.

Tim suspected the worst. He had done reasonably well until the last question, when he had run out of time. 'I only wrote two sides of A4 on it and, unless I packed it with facts, that won't be enough.' Angela and Emily were anxious, but as they heard the reactions of others around them, began to think that they might have done well enough after all. Corinne was uncertain.

The usual post-exam cries of 'I'm sure I've failed' had more substance to them this time round. Many people were seriously worried. The habitual low-key criticism of the college swelled into something louder and more heartfelt as students complained that they should have received better preparation for the exam.

For those who failed, the implications would be serious.

They would have to resit the exam in September, only weeks before the final exam of the course was due to take place. Inevitably, studying for the resits would leave them less time to study for this final exam. Yet they wouldn't be able to skimp on revision: you were allowed only two attempts at each exam: anyone who failed the resit would be off the course, even at this late stage.

Not everyone thought this would be such a bad thing. Jane was feeling fed up with the course anyway. The branch hadn't lived up to her hopes so far: she hadn't enjoyed working with the other staff on the wards and didn't feel that she had learnt very much. She certainly didn't feel that she was 'a real nurse'. She was beginning to panic that she was training for the wrong career and was tempted to give up. These days she tended to get away from the hospital and the nurses' home in her free hours; she was spending a lot of time with a very close friend, Stephen, whom she had met before starting the course and who was also a Buddhist. She was hard to get hold of, but reports of her state of mind filtered back to me.

'She's very fed up,' Angela said. 'We're all saying to her: "Hold on, you've got this far; hang on till the end of the course." '

At this stage, despite her own advice, Angela was inclined to share Jane's disillusionment. She had enjoyed her first rostered service placement (on an acute surgery ward at the Wavetree) more than she had expected. But she still felt that nurses were undervalued and underpaid, and chafed at the lack of autonomy. She was grimly determined to finish the course and register, all the same.

By contrast, the other adult branch students, Emily, Tim and Corinne, were enjoying their work and were still very much committed to nursing. They had no desire at all to leave the course. They did their best to put their anxieties on one side until the results came out (expected in mid-July); they were helped by the prospect of new placements.

Tim was going on to a renal (kidney) ward; Emily on to ENT (Ear, Nose and Throat). Corinne was starting cardiology. Jane was to go (somewhat reluctantly) on to a general medical ward at the Wavetree and Angela would start work on an oncology ward at Alf's, which specialized in radiotherapy. In fact, Angela was quietly dreading this placement; her best friend had died of cancer since she had been in England, and she was afraid that the associations would be too strong for her.

More happily, Rachel had learnt that she was to go back to Howard for the summer. And Nicola had elected to do a community-based placement for the next three months. She had made the choice with one eye firmly on career prospects: 'We've got to do one long placement in the community and one in an institution before the end of the course. I thought I'd prefer to be doing the institutional one towards the end, as I'll be starting to look for jobs then and I think there's probably a better chance of finding one on a ward.'

Her community placement was to be at the Link, a day centre based in St Wenceslas' Hospital, which ran therapeutic groups. Coincidentally, she was not the only nurse in this book who started work there in July.

CATHERINE FORD'S year had been very up and down so far. Missing out on the CPN job at the start of the year had shaken her badly, but once she had recovered from the shock, she had actually felt much better about staying on Wilcox, the acute mental health ward. 'It pulled me up and made me assess myself. I asked myself what I wanted to do and what I *could* do, and I realized that all right, I didn't get that job, but I do have an awful lot to offer. And that's made me feel very positive. I decided that as I was staying on Wilcox, I'd give my very best to the work. And after that I really enjoyed it.'

But although work was satisfying, she felt at low ebb

personally. Her health wasn't good: 'I've had some kind of post-viral thing and I've been very tired. I think I've shaken it off now, but it's been pulling me down.'

Listening to Catherine talk, it's hard to gauge how far she is responding to external factors, such as physical illness and the demands of work, and how much of the pressure springs from within. She finds it quite hard to know, too.

Certainly, although she had a good relationship with Bob, their circumstances weren't ideal: they were often doing opposite shifts and couldn't spend as much time together as they wanted. Getting leave together was also difficult. Catherine's main holiday for this year wasn't going to be with Bob: she had booked to go to the Caribbean with her mother in June.

At the beginning of June she got an unexpected telephone call from the manager of the Link. The manager said that he'd heard Catherine was interested in going into the community. The Link was accounted a community resource and there was a vacancy for a staff nurse: would she be interested in applying?

Catherine might have put conscious thoughts of leaving Wilcox out of her mind, but a nagging sense that she really ought to be making a move now rushed to the surface and proved hard to ignore. Curious to know more about the Link, she filled in the application form and went for an interview.

The Link is housed in the basement of St Wenceslas' central, red-brick block. It is a grim site but the Link itself is nicely decorated inside and has a relaxed but efficient atmosphere. It had been founded four years previously, as a development of the work done in St Wenceslas' occupational therapy department. It draws its clients from the community of Wavetree; they can be referred to the Link by acute mental health wards (including Wilcox), by GPs, by social services or by themselves – they can simply turn up and ask to be considered for treatment. The Link offers group work of various kinds (from assertiveness to drama therapy groups, from relaxation to women's and men's discussion groups) and each client has a programme of groups worked out to meet his or her needs. The people who come to the Link are clients, not patients: they come because they want to and go home again afterwards. The groups operate on an eight-week cycle and ideally one cycle will be enough to help clients start to address their problems more independently; if not, they can return for a second cycle and – in rare circumstances – they might come back for a third.

There was one feature of the Link which immediately appealed to Catherine: 'The power base is with the nurses, which is very unusual. As you know, that's often been a bugbear of mine on the wards.'

A team of nurses runs the Link. True, there is a consultant psychiatrist attached to the place and every client entering a programme will be seen once by him or another doctor; the consultant also has weekly 'ward rounds' when he meets the nurses and discusses their concerns about particular clients. But the groups are devised and run by the nurses; the nurses assess all the clients and decide who to take on to the programme and who to refer elsewhere. And the 'ward rounds' with the consultant are led by the nurses too: it is they who put forward clients and situations for discussion.

When Catherine was shown round, Holly, the ward manager, was on maternity leave, but she met the rest of the full-time team: John (the charge nurse) and two staff nurses, Helen and Roberta. Holly and Roberta had both been there since the beginning and from what she heard Catherine was left in no doubt that Holly was an assertive woman who had fought to make the Link nurse-led and autonomous of the hospital.

Catherine was not sure how she would get on with Holly in person, but she felt that here was a good opportunity to widen her experience and move with the tide into the community. On the other hand it would be a very structured way of working, which she wasn't used to; she had little experience in running groups, and she would be working nine to five, five days a week, and therefore losing all her (not inconsiderable) unsocial hours pay.

When she was offered the job, soon afterwards, she couldn't make up her mind. She talked it over with her colleagues on Wilcox, particularly Malcolm. He told her it would be a good move for her and she should take it; they would always have her back on Wilcox if it didn't work out. Catherine knew he was right but felt reluctant to leave the safety of Wilcox; all the same, she felt that she would have to accept the offer or be considered indecisive. She bought a bit of time by asking if she could give her decision when she returned from holiday.

The holiday should have been wonderful. Catherine and her mother went to Margarita, an island off the coast of Venezuela, with beautiful beaches and not too much development. However, they stayed in the capital town, which they found dirty and noisy. Catherine's mother was mugged. And when she got back to England, Catherine felt distinctly unrefreshed. Perhaps, she acknowledged afterwards, it was tension about the impending move that had made everything seem so difficult. Whatever the reason, she was already rather overwrought when she accepted the Link's offer and gave in her official notice at Wilcox.

As the Link needed her quickly, for the beginning of July, Wilcox asked her to work just two weeks' notice. She would rather have gone at once: speaking to me after the first 'last' week, she said she was finding it very hard. 'I don't want to engage with the fact that I'm leaving. I'm really struggling with it. I'm getting very tearful and feel very attached to it. And I've still got to do good work here, with the patients. I'm dreading all the goodbyes.'

But she survived them, as people do. Her colleagues held

a party for her and gave her a present. She cried, promised to keep in touch, and the following Monday started work at the Link.

It was week six of the current eight-week programme, so Catherine had a few weeks' grace before she had to start running groups herself. The time was given over to studying how the Link operated, learning how to assess new clients and taking on a small caseload of people for whom she would be primary nurse.

The Link ran groups only three days a week. Monday was assessment day, when prospective clients came along to be interviewed and assessed. Groups met on Tuesday, Wednesday and Thursday. On these days the Link was also open for clients to drop in, chat to one another and have meetings with their primary nurses. On Friday, some individual work was done between staff and their key clients. Friday was also staff supervision day: the staff spent the time in formal interviews with their supervisors, assessing their own work, and in informal discussions with one another about the way the programme was going and other management matters. Once a fortnight a group analyst came in, to discuss the group work with the nurses.

This high level of supervision was very rare for psychiatric nursing and, Catherine felt, very valuable. It certainly helped her during her weeks of induction when she was building up a client list and trying to learn about the group work. In fact, she relied totally on staff discussion for information about the groups: the Link operated a closed group policy which meant that once the group had met twice, no one new could join it or sit in on it. This protected the clients from feeling exposed or disrupted, but made it impossible for Catherine to get any first-hand experience of the groups before running some.

Having sat in on several assessments and conducted a few herself under supervision, Catherine now began to do her own. She ended up admitting five people and became their primary nurse for the programme ahead.

They were: Elizabeth, a woman in her mid-forties whose son had recently died of leukaemia and who was now suffering panic attacks and agoraphobia; Danny, a young man who had hit his partner a few times and who was terrified of becoming habitually violent; Teresa, a young woman who had been sexually abused as a child and who had been suffering panic attacks since she had had her own baby, eight months before; Ilana, an isolated young woman who had recently moved to England and whose father had died; and Felicity, who was in a bad relationship with her partner and wanted to become more assertive.

Of all of these, Catherine had most doubts about Felicity. 'She referred herself here, because she's a very anxious young woman. She's in a relationship with a partner – it's fairly abusive really. She's thinking of settling down with him and she knows it's not ideal – she's worried about it. She's got an awful problem with self-esteem. She's got no confidence and she finds it difficult to assert herself. These are the areas she wants to work at.

'Now there is one thing we have to take into consideration when we assess people: everyone who comes on to a programme here sees a psychiatrist and it goes on their medical records. They acquire a psychiatric history, and that can have implications for them. You are often supposed to declare it if you're applying for jobs, for instance, or on insurance forms.

'I said to her, "Well, this is the score. I feel quite strongly that it would be a shame for you to get a psychiatric record." I suggested two services in the community she could go to; and the local college of education is running an assertiveness course. And she could go along to Relate of course. But she was very keen to come to the Link. So she's going to come on the next programme – just to the assertiveness groups, because she works. And I'll probably see her about three times, to talk over how it's going.'

Barely a week after Catherine started work there, Nicola arrived at the Link. As fellow newcomers, they were learning together and within a few days they discovered that I'd been talking to them both. 'So much for confidentiality!' Catherine said accusingly.

They also shared a supervisor: John, the charge nurse. He had been at the Link two years and was currently doing a drama therapy course, which he was using in his work. He made an immediate impression on both of them.

'He's very psychodynamic in his approach,' said Catherine. 'He thinks like a therapist rather than a nurse, he's very flexible. When I came back after the first few days I thought, "Wow! Well, I've got to have a male hero to worship and I'm worshipping John." Last time I saw Malcolm I told him he'd been usurped.'

'He's very, very skilled and I'm learning a lot from him,' said Nicola, somewhat less emotionally.

There was another student at the Link too, but she was on the RGN course and doing only a brief placement. She did not get as involved as Nicola, who from the outset was finding the Link a stimulating place to work.

'She's a very motivated young woman,' said Catherine, remarking on the fact that Nicola had asked to sit in on a whole range of groups when the new programme began. Like the other permanent staff, she was impressed by Nicola's commitment and her appetite for learning. She was also a touch envious: 'In a sense we're learning together – but of course she won't be expected to actually run the groups.'

Catherine, by contrast, was assigned seven groups to run on the new programme. Some she would take in partnership with another nurse, some alone. She was apprehensive as the first sessions approached and rather cross about the lack of guidance. 'I've been given relaxation groups to run alone – two practice groups, which seem to be the ones novices always get given, and a relaxation theory group. They just said,

"That's yours." I've never sat in on one even and I'm doing this alone. It's ridiculous.'

She would also be co-running four groups, two with Roberta: time management, a fairly formal teaching group which would help clients suffering from anxiety to use their time, and expression, a more open-ended discussion-style group. These had never been run before and it would be up to Catherine and Roberta to devise an approach for them.

The groups which Catherine would be helping to run with Helen were well established: assertiveness and a women's group, again a formal 'teaching' group and an unstructured group respectively. 'Helen's been doing the assertiveness groups for a long time, so I think that'll be fairly straightforward. It's the two new groups I'm anxious about. Mind you, I'm anxious about anything at the moment.'

The first sessions of the relaxation groups allayed her fears somewhat. The practice sessions went well, with Catherine using a script to lead the physical relaxing exercises, and she approached the theory in an unformalized, discussion-based way, exploring the physiology of relaxation and the problems that can interfere with it. The clients seemed interested and responded well.

The first meeting of the time management group, however, was less successful. The group was aimed at people suffering from anxiety and depression, who found it difficult to structure their time. The inability to use time, or to get things done, is a common symptom of these conditions. People feel, as Catherine put it, 'that they don't count for anything', and they stop being able to cope with the routine transactions of daily life. Unfortunately, going along to the Link is one of these transactions and on the first day only two of the eight enrolled clients turned up.

'And they didn't want to talk about time management – they wanted to talk about their problems! One of them said time management wasn't a problem for him at all; he could write a book on it. In fact, he could run a group on it. It was just that at the moment he was so obsessed with his major problems he couldn't even get out of bed in the morning. And he knew that if he could just sort his problems out and become less depressed, he could manage his time. He was more or less saying, 'I don't think this is pertinent for me to come into.' So I said we valued his contribution and perhaps he could share some of his expertise with the group! And I pointed out that although he said he couldn't get out of bed in the morning, he'd come for the group so it had performed a function for him already. He went, 'Oh, yeah.'

'The other guy said that the reason he couldn't manage his time was that he was depressed and couldn't cope with meeting people.

'It was difficult. In the end we brainstormed about time management and the problems people have with it, and then we had planned to get the clients into groups of two to look at possible ways of managing time. So the two of them talked about it a bit and worked out some objectives for themselves. Then we gave them each a timetable to go away with. They'll fill it in and bring it back next week, to show what they've done with their week.'

Meanwhile, Catherine and Roberta would call around the other clients and try to get a better turn out for the second session. Catherine felt that however many people came, it was going to be a tricky group. 'I can't quite see how it's going to shape, so far. The trouble is, they want to talk about their problems rather than time management, and the problems they express are going to be very disparate.'

She didn't feel completely at ease with Roberta, either. In many ways she admired her: Roberta had begun her career as an enrolled nurse, gone into psychiatry and worked at Wilcox, then the Link, and had now completed a conversion course and become a registered mental nurse. But her approach to the groups differed from Catherine's: 'She's more structured than me and I'm worried that she'll be a stickler for rules. I don't like to be too regimented. To my view, if things can be done another way and it might work, I'll do it.'

In fact, Catherine was relieved to find that within the group they worked together well. But she found these early weeks at the Link a terrible strain: she often went home so tired that her head ached and it would be an hour or two before she could think straight. She felt that she had jumped into the unknown by coming here and she kept waiting to be told that her face did not fit.

For Nicola, meanwhile, being at the Link was almost unalloyed pleasure. After her growing disillusionment with care in the community, based on what she had seen with the CPN, it was a relief to be able to immerse herself in a small community-based unit which really did seem to work. 'I don't think it's particularly well funded but it's cost-effective because it runs time-limited courses. People come into a very focused programme for eight weeks and attend groups which are felt to be specifically suited to their problems.'

As the new programme progressed, Nicola was busy getting involved with a wide range of groups. She deliberately tried to take part in as many as possible. 'They divide up in three ways really. There are basically teaching groups, which are structured, have an agenda, they're safer groups really for people to come into as they're almost like classes. They are assertiveness, stress management, time management, relaxation and interpersonal skills. There are other unstructured talking groups; they are men's group, a women's group and awareness – which is traditional group therapy. Then there's drama therapy, which is a combination of the two – it's planned, but open for people to interpret the plan using creative means to express feelings and confront problems.'

Drama therapy was John's group, and so one of the ones Nicola attended regularly. 'As John's my mentor, I'm sort of helping to run his groups. I'm not an actual facilitator but I'm there and I can contribute.'

Contributing to the drama therapy turned out to be something of a challenge for her. 'It was all new for me and I was very uncomfortable at first because it's not my sort of thing. It's all about creative expression – for instance, you might write, or draw, or you might use a body costume to sculpt a feeling. I was embarrassed. For certain people who find it hard to verbalize and for creative people, who express things in a creative way, it's good.'

Much more up Nicola's street were the groups which centred around verbal communication, like assertiveness, awareness and the women's group. John ran the awareness group, together with Tracey, an outside assistant. Nicola was fascinated by the skill John showed in this group and perturbed in equal measure by what she considered Tracey's overbearing approach. 'I actually think she's dreadful, but unfortunately she's been doing this group for yonks. She's terribly directive and confrontational with people who are often quite fragile and nervous and it seems that everything is your mother's fault or your parents' fault. She doesn't *offer* interpretations; it's "You're like this because your mother did this to you." And I'm thinking, you don't know this person! You've just met them for goodness sake!

'She interrupts people, doesn't let them finish their sentence, monopolizes time. The other week I came out fuming! John's a good balance to her, but I don't understand how he keeps working with her.'

Some members of the group dropped out after a few sessions – a common phenomenon, as group therapy can be daunting and is often painful. One of these was Michael, a university student who had attempted suicide. Nicola was his primary nurse and she struggled to keep him involved.

'He's a lovely bloke. He took sixty paracetemol and had liver damage, which meant he was six weeks on a ward. They referred him to the Link when he was discharged, but really the Link wasn't suitable for him. I encouraged him to come to the groups but his attendance was always erratic and when he came he'd just clam up. I'd see him one to one, but often he'd call me and make an appointment and then not turn up. You can get people concerned in you by being vocal and visible, or by being the complete opposite, and that's what he was doing.'

Nicola felt protective towards Michael and did her best to keep in touch, but she and the other staff recognized that the Link, which requires a certain amount of independent motivation from its clients, couldn't give Michael what he needed. He was referred on for psychotherapy in the community, and Nicola took some comfort from the fact that he would be monitored by his psychotherapist. 'At least he's safe.'

She was also primary nurse to Victor, who was attending almost every group going at the Link, including awareness and Catherine and Roberta's time management. Victor was a lonely man in his forties, who had lived with his mother and some of his sisters until his mother's recent death. The mother had been a dominating figure who had brought her children up to believe that men were always trying to get sex from women. Victor had taken this to heart and struggled to live with what he felt must be dirty and predatory sexual desires. He didn't have friends outside the family and found it impossible to form a relationship with a woman because, as he said in the men's group: 'If you ask a woman out, she'll think you want sex.' He had been to prostitutes a few times, which had reinforced his low opinion of himself.

Since his mother had died, Victor could no longer cope with living with his sisters and had moved out, to live alone. He was very depressed and had been visiting his mother's grave two or three times a day; recently he had begun to hear her voice during these visits, criticizing him. Lonely, guilty and afraid, he had eventually walked into Wavetree Casualty and they had referred him here.

When Nicola assessed him, he was 'a bag of nerves. He was so lonely and missed his mother so much. And he felt guilty about everything. He was worried that she would tell him off when he died, and he said that she was calling him from the grave and criticizing him for coming to the Link.'

Victor knew that he wasn't really hearing his mother's voice (he had what the mental health profession calls 'insight') but he couldn't stop imagining it and being tormented by it. Once he began on his intensive and time-consuming programme of groups, however, he made steady progress. Despite telling Catherine at the first time management session that he couldn't cope with meeting people, he found that he enjoyed the contact with the other clients and he would come all three days every week, attend the groups, chat to clients and staff and have regular one-to-one talks with Nicola. The staff were all pleased to see his progress: both Catherine and Nicola were fond of him, Catherine describing him as 'a real sweetie' and Nicola as 'one of my favourite clients'. The only problem was that he began to grow dependent on Nicola.

'He's thinking of me a lot; he says like a brother. He's worried about my safety and he says how nice I am because I've listened to him. He's upset because I'm going to leave. I'm sad for him because I didn't want this to happen and I worked hard to prevent it but perhaps it's inevitable – this is probably the first relationship where someone has listened to him.'

Half way through the programme, Nicola described herself as being 'on a high'. She felt that she was learning a huge amount from the courses, and particularly from the way that John worked with clients.

'One of the people in the awareness group is Simon,

who's in his fifties and used to have a business that failed. His business values were the way he validated himself: through wealth, achievements, respect from other business people. He's had two broken marriages and now that his business is gone he believes he'll never find another woman unless he's solvent again. He sank into a depression about it all.

'He has been challenged in the group about how much he harps on about the past and how unrealistic his goals are. He thinks he's worthless unless he's a millionaire and he used to bore people silly with financial details about his business and what happened to it. Gradually his barriers have been breaking down (it's been fascinating to watch) and one day he said that he wanted guidance from the group. John said, "All we can do is feed back what you say and our views." And the views that came out were that he was a difficult person; he tended to push away other people's observations and defend himself as if he was being attacked; and that he was always proving himself.

'He was stunned. He had no idea that was how he was seen. The next week he suddenly began talking about his father: he told us that his father had never validated him and he'd always had to prove himself. That's the kind of thing that can happen in a group when you've got someone with John's skill.'

Unfortunately, shortly after this Nicola's exhilaration was dealt a blow by some bad news from home: her father was seriously ill. The business of the Link dwindled rapidly in importance. For the next few weeks, Nicola was stretched very thin: she put in her five-day weeks at the Link, phoned home every evening and at weekends she travelled the 200 miles to be with her father and take some of the strain off her mother. At work she was preoccupied with her anxiety for him and found it hard to concentrate on the groups and the clients: 'It's partly that my mind is all over the place but partly it's that you start thinking, "Well, I've got problems too." '

Being able to air her feelings in supervisions helped, but what Nicola really wanted was to take some time off and go home. She asked her course tutor if it could be arranged and suggested that she defer taking the October exams until winter, when she could take them along with resit candidates. The response from the college was that if she wanted time out, she should take six months and do the final exams and placements with the next lot of Project 2000 students. The idea dismayed her. Her parents were anxious that she shouldn't disrupt her training so she decided to stay on and go home whenever she could manage. But she continued her campaign to postpone taking the exam, as she wasn't able to concentrate properly on her reading.

In the meantime, Catherine was feeling calmer and more confident. She was still very tired, very often, but she was now inclined to put this down to the post-viral syndrome, which she suspected might be still hanging round. She did not feel the same acute stress as before; in fact she and her clients were learning to relax together.

Catherine's own special clients were making varying degrees of progress. Felicity (whom she'd had doubts about taking) was making the most of the assertiveness group and had justified her own insistence that she come to the Link. 'She does really well; she takes things on board and gets a lot from it. She's going to be discharged at the end of the programme and I'm giving her a list of counsellors in the community. She wants someone to talk to and this really isn't the right place for her.' The only problem was that Felicity might have trouble being taken on by anyone in the NHS now: 'She really isn't unwell enough.'

Danny, the young man who had hit his partner, was likewise someone who didn't really have mental health problems. But the difficulties he was experiencing in close relationships were severe enough, and the propensity to violence worrying enough, for him to have been accepted into several groups.

'He's doing stress management, relaxation and a talking group, where he can express a lot of things. And we've had one-to-one sessions together. I don't feel judgemental about him – I think I would if he was an absolute pig, that would only be human, but he's a lovely man and it's all to do with things from his childhood and he's really, really mortified. He carries it around like a cross and feels terrible. He's separated from his partner now but really wants to make a new relationship with her. He perceives it all as his problem and some of the work I've been doing has been to show that it's not. It's to do with the relationship and the way she responds to him.' Catherine also concentrated on helping Danny with practical things, like incorporating relaxation techniques into his life. Danny would not be re-enrolled on the next programme, but he would be attending the year-long support group that was being set up for former clients.

Elizabeth, the woman whose son had died, was attending the Link while she was on the waiting list for psychotherapy. She was often very angry and, as she learnt more of Elizabeth's life, Catherine was not surprised. 'She was abused sexually as a young woman and hates men. She finds it very difficult to be with men – she gets upset at the smell of them, she says. In the mixed groups she has to sit with women. The only man of any significance was her son and now he's gone. She had a very close relationship with him: he sounds lovely and was apparently very talented, he won all these prizes at school. He took his A levels just before he died and after his death the results came out and they were very good.

'As time passes she says something more, happens to drop in some new, awful piece of her history and you think, my God, what sort of life have you had?'

Teresa, who had an eight-month-old daughter, had also been sexually abused in the past. She'd had a previous spate of panic attacks and had got over them, with help from the charity Childline. But since the birth of her baby they had returned; she lived in dread of something bad happening to the child and at night, instead of sleeping, she sat up, watching the baby's breathing. At first she had not managed to come to many of the groups, nor to many sessions with Catherine, due to a mixture of childminding problems and her own anxiety. However, she was attending fairly regularly now and would be coming again to the next programme.

Ilana had come to this country from abroad, where she had lived with her father till his recent death. She was suffering anxiety and depression; she was isolated at home living with her mother and had few friends in London. She made periodic appearances at the women's group where she 'never says a thing'. However, she assured Catherine that she did get something out of it, and it was arranged that she should attend some of the more structured groups next time round.

At the beginning of the programme, Catherine had been by no means sure that *she* would still be here next time around. But now, as her nervousness decreased and John continued to assure her in supervisions that she was doing well, she thought that after all she might make a go of it here.

TIM WAS HAPPILY making a go of his summer placement on Fairbrother renal ward at Alf's. He considered himself lucky to have gone there straight from the Markham Hospital: not only were they both 'speciality' placements, where the nurses were highly skilled and quite powerful, but both offered a mixture of surgical and medical work. In the Markham, patients with chronic conditions like Crohn's and ulcerative colitis had come in to be treated with medication and/or surgery. On Fairbrother, people with chronic kidney failure would be admitted for dialysis and, in some cases, for transplants. Tim would be working on the medical side, in the twenty-two-bed ward, but he would be able to follow the progress of patients admitted for transplants, and he might be able to see some minor surgical procedures.

'I prefer surgery to medicine, probably for selfish reasons. I like to see people come into hospital, have their operation, get better and go home.' He would not be seeing permanent cures on Fairbrother but he would be learning about the extraordinary difference made to people's lives by good dialysis.

The kidneys perform many functions: they regulate the body's fluid levels, get rid of harmful products from the bloodstream and help the bones absorb calcium. When they start to fail the patient suffers high blood pressure, fluid retention and anaemia, along with a host of unpleasant side effects such as nausea, itching and confusion. If untreated, kidney failure will eventually kill.

The most common way of treating renal failure is dialysis: this used always to mean haemodialysis, when the patient is attached to a heavy and expensive machine which filters all the blood in the body. The process is efficient but takes several hours and patients usually have to undergo it two or three times a week. On the floor below Fairbrother Ward is Alf's haemodialysis ward: a large room in which each bed is accompanied by its own unwieldy machine. Patients book themselves in for regular sessions: some come in overnight and go off to work the next day; others sit reading or lie drowsing as the machines do their slow and thorough job. Approximately eighty patients a week come to Alf's for regular haemodialysis.

There is now another kind of dialysis avilable, however. Known as CAPD (Continuous Ambulatory Peritoneal Dialysis), it can be done by the patients themselves, requires no machine and is portable. It works rather like the Hickman line. A soft plastic tube called a Tenckhoff catheter is surgically inserted in the abdomen, with two ends emerging. The patient then screws a bag of dialysing fluid on to the 'in' end, and an empty bag to the 'out' end. The bag of dialysing fluid is hooked to a small stand higher than the patient's abdomen and then by gravity the fluid flows down through the peritoneum and flushes harmful products from the blood. The process doesn't hurt though there is a slight sensation of pressure; it takes half an hour and must usually be done three times a day.

It's fair to say that CAPD really has revolutionized the lives of many people with renal failure. It frees them from coming into hospital for haemodialysis; it allows them to live normal lives, to have jobs, to go to college. From the NHS's point of view, it also wins by being cheaper than traditional haemodialysis. However, it requires a good level of knowledge from the patient, close monitoring and an understanding of the dangers of infection. A fairly large part of the work in Alf's renal unit now involves training patients in the use of CAPD and showing them how to monitor themselves for possible problems. On average one hundred patients come to the unit every week with some kind of CAPD problem. The majority are minor problems, such as slight water retention or dehydration, which can be treated by adjusting treatment and/or diet. Some are more serious: any hint of an infection in the peritoneum spells danger, and patients showing suspicious symptoms are immediately admitted.

At the end of two weeks, Tim knew his way around the ward, was settling in to his alloted place in one of the four nursing teams and had got to know some of the patients. 'The youngest is fifteen, the oldest is eighty-two. About half of them are diabetic: renal failure is one of the side effects of diabetes. It's not a definite but there's a higher incidence of it later in life, for people who've been diabetic a long time.

'Diabetes is horrible. It can affect your eyes, so if you can't see well and you develop chronic renal failure, then you can't have CAPD, because changing the bag's a sterile technique and you wouldn't be able to see well enough to do it. So quite a few of our diabetic patients are on haemodialysis. Some have had amputations as well – that's because diabetes affects the circulation and people can get gangrene in their limbs.'

There was one woman who seemed to Tim to sum up the ravages of a lifetime of diabetes. 'She's had both legs amputated and also she's unfortunately had quite a lot of bowel removed. She's got a stoma and she wants to stop treatment. She doesn't want to continue with dialysis, she just wants to die. But her husband's really upset and wants her to carry on.

'She's not old at all – she's only forty-three. And from the hips down she's got no legs at all. She only came in yesterday, but she's quite a regular patient. A lot of the staff are quite sad to see her: last time she had one leg left, this time she's got no legs; she's going blind, she's on quite a lot of pain control. She doesn't see a future for herself. If it wasn't for the husband she would just say, "End the treatment" and we would.'

It was impossible for the nurses to do anything for this woman other than give her pain relief and some measure of human comfort. For most of the patients, though, the outlook was much better. Quite a few were having Tenckhoff catheters inserted and were being trained in the use of CAPD. The operation itself was simple and done under local anaesthetic, but because the risk of infection was very high, the nursing care required afterwards was intensive.

'A lot of my work is doing observations, especially blood pressure. Straight after theatre, patients are checked every five to ten minutes. Then after an hour or so, it goes down to once every half an hour, then once every hour. When they are no longer acute, they are checked four times a day.

'I'm also now allowed to changed dressings on the catheter site. Post-surgery they have to be changed every day for the first ten days and then every two days. The way they do it on the ward here is the way they train the patients to do it, so every nurse has to do it exactly the same so as not to confuse the patients. It's strange: normally when you're doing an aseptic dressing, you're very careful about where you put things. But when you're doing it here, you just drop things on the floor then you pick them up at the end. I found that hard at first. Take the dressing from the wound, drop it on the floor, clean the wound, drop the gauze on the floor . . . it is quite strange. But now I quite enjoy it!'

Tim developed more skills as the placement went on. He found it a good ward on which to learn. The nurses had great expertise and the doctors treated them with respect – or most doctors did. 'I've grown to respect the doctors, mostly. Though there are some junior ones (senior medical students are the worst) who are very jumped up and think they know a lot more than they do. And the other day I saw a senior registrar removing sutures from a patient: afterwards he actually left the cutter on the patient's bed. And I went up to him and said, "Excuse me, that's sharp. You're supposed to dispose of sharps. Would you mind doing so?" Nurses don't normally do that – they clean up after the doctor. And he looked at me as if I was mad – "Who do you think you're talking to?" But he knew I was right and did it. He could have said sorry though.'

There were no such problems with the nursing staff. Susan, the sister on Fairbrother, was good at teaching students while allowing them to work at their own pace. She encouraged Tim to get around and see different aspects of the unit: he was planning a day down on haemodialysis, and on the day I was there Susan told him that if he wanted to see a nurse training a patient to use CAPD, there would be an opportunity that afternoon.

Her attitude, confident and reasonably relaxed, applied to the patients as well. This was important, as many of them were on the ward for weeks as a time. They were able to set their own routine, within the limits of what the ward could manage; for the smokers among them this meant regular trips on to the cast-iron fire escape to smoke in the pallid city sunshine.

Tim felt that he fitted into the team well. He regretted not being able to nurse the transplant patients, but they were put in individual side rooms and their nurses kept to a minimum because they were vulnerable to infection immediately after the operation.

He developed some useful skills with the other patients though: 'I took out some staples yesterday. They staple people now rather than stitch them, it leaves a smaller scar. The patient was scared – they're always scared about the staples, even when they've had a massive operation – and she said: "Have you ever done this before?" And I said, "No, but I used to work in a stationer's so don't worry!" She said, "I'm really nervous," so I said, "Sing." And so we sang all the way through it. I had them out before she even realized it.'

In the middle of July, the adult branch exam results came out. They were worse than anyone had expected: two thirds of the group had failed. There was consternation in the college and panic amongst the students. Questions were raised about the marking methods used and in a flurry of activity, many of the failed papers were passed to moderators for re-examination.

On first marking, Tim, Corinne and Jane had all failed. When the papers came back from the moderator, there was good news for Tim. 'The moderator marked me up by ten marks on one question, which I'd failed. The original marker said I was obviously widely read in the subject – I'd quoted several research studies as reasons for doing things – but then on his mark for research and rationale, he wrote nought. The moderator looked at the paper and said the marker's comments were right, so why weren't they reflected in the mark? The extra marks put me up beyond the pass level.'

The moderator marked up twenty of the failed students in all, so that eventually only one-third of the group faced resits. But one-third was still a high proportion. And many of the marked-up students felt unhappy: whose judgement should they rely on, that of the original marker or the moderator? The original marker had been a tutor from Alf's, which hardly encouraged confidence in the course.

Corinne and Jane were among the remaining third who failed. Jane had always known she would have to resit, after her early exit from the paper. Corinne was shaken, though she took comfort from the fact that so many were in the same situation. The resit loomed uncompromisingly ahead. We were due to meet at the end of July, but she rang up and cancelled: she was going to see her tutor instead, to discuss what she should study between now and September. She sounded slightly flustered and said that for the next few weeks she would be concentrating on work; I promised to stay out of her way till the resit was over.

The resit candidates had to study in such spare time as they could find from their ward work. The placements were due to run until late September, and students wanting changes to their off duty for whatever reasons – holiday, revision, personal crisis – had to put their requests to the sister or ward manager in charge and hope for the best. The permanent staff were usually ready to help, but they couldn't always negotiate their way round staffing crises or a particularly heavy time on the ward.

Jane was currently on Landor, a general medical ward at Wavetree. They had all sorts of patients there: 'Anything and everything. Quite a lot of people with leg ulcers, alcoholics, diabetics, suicides, old people that have fallen down.' Like most general medical wards, it was hard work, but she was finally enjoying herself. She liked the nurses and especially the ward manager: 'I really respect her,' she said, with an air of surprise. She also liked the fact that the ward was a ten-minute walk from her room, so she could have an extra half-hour in bed before each shift and still be certain to be on time.

Angela was having a more challenging time. It should have been a pleasant summer for her: she had passed the exam and her term of office as chair of the Students' Representative Council had now ended. This was a huge relief. as often happens with these things, it was only once it was over that she realised how much time and energy it had involved.

But at home things were difficult. Her husband, Mark, had not got on as well as he'd hoped in theatrical design, and the fact that he was in his late thirties had suddenly started to anguish him. 'He's going through some kind of mid-life crisis,' Angela said, not entirely humorously. ' "What have I achieved in my life? Where am I going?" Oh God.'

An old friend of his had just asked if he'd be interested in going into business with him, in America. Mark wanted to do it, so they agreed that he would go in August. Angela would join him nine months later, as soon as she finished her training.

She was dreading the separation. She was also cast down by the prospect of giving up the flat (she wouldn't be able to afford it alone) and moving into one of the nurses' homes.

Meanwhile, she had her summer placement on Friedricks oncology ward to deal with. It was two years since her friend had died, but Angela had not been able to get home, either during the last illness or for the funeral, and so she hadn't even begun to come to terms with the loss. She was still grieving and afraid that she wouldn't be able to cope with patients suffering the same kinds of illness.

The oncology wards in Alf's had a good reputation for looking after their staff, so on her first day Angela approached the sister and explained the background to her worries. She had been expecting some guidance, perhaps some practical suggestions about getting emotional support. Instead, 'Never mind,' said the sister. Not knowing what to make of this most English of responses, Angela feared the worst: 'I felt almost that by asking for support, I was going to get less than had I not. I almost branded myself.'

In the event, however, there was a good deal of support for staff, both formal (there were group meetings and a counsellor available) and more generally, in a spirit of comradeship amongst the nurses.

There are two oncology wards at Alf's: Preston, which specialises in blood cancers (and where Emily had begun rostered service) and Friedricks. Friedricks treats the range of cancers but specializes in radiotherapy. Radiotherapy is used typically on brain cancers, lung cancers and secondaries where the cancer has gone into metastasis (spread from one part of the body to another). It is also used for other forms of cancer, in cases where the cancer is difficult to treat surgically, and as part of a combination of treatments, together with chemotherapy and/or surgery.

As on Preston, the patients came in when first diagnosed and then returned, at different intervals and for different lengths of stay, to have courses of treatment. It is not always a clear-cut decision whether a cancer should be treated with chemotherapy or radiotherapy; in these cases the doctors often prescribe both ('adjunct therapy').

Because the care is highly specialized, and a matter of life and death, the student nurse's role in it is limited. As Emily had found on Preston, much of it consisted of doing observations and then liaising with one of the registered nurses. The situation was exacerbated by what Angela thought was a proprietorial relationship between some nurses and their patients: 'They rather keep their patients to themselves, as if they owned this and that patient. There isn't much team work going on and the feeling on the ward is divided. I don't feel part of a team and I don't think the other students do – you're told you can do something one day and the next you're told you can't do it. There isn't really any remit for having students on the ward. This is something we get all the time, but I think here they're particularly uptight. I think perhaps it's in the nature of oncology.'

One thing Angela was allowed to do was talk to patients at length and she gradually came to realize that this forms a large part of oncology nursing, no matter what grade a nurse is.

'Radiotherapy is odd – it's not invasive in any way and it's not painful, but there are these big machines and I think it's hard for patients to see that it's actually doing anything, because they don't see anything or feel anything. With chemotherapy, at least you have a needle in the arm and this bag and these drugs.

'You give information pre-treatment. And like chemotherapy, radiotherapy has side effects – nausea, vomiting, skin reactions, hair loss, swelling, double vision. So you treat those. But mostly I think it's helping them see that something is being done for them.'

Many people came in for radiotherapy as outpatients, so on the days that Angela was attached to the radiotherapy department itself she saw people who were actually quite well. The shifts that she worked on the ward were different: many of the people there were very sick indeed and several died during her placement.

Like Emily before her, Angela became deeply interested in the process of dying. 'It's not that you're alive one moment and dead the next. People go in and out of consciousness and you can almost see that they're not really in their bodies any more. It's interesting and fascinating and I'm really glad I got the chance to deal with it.'

Being with people while they died did not come easily to her; whereas Emily had followed her instincts, talking to those who could hear, stroking the hands of those who couldn't understand, Angela was never sure what to do. 'When they're in the very last throes of leaving this life, they're not speaking any more, there's very little eye contact... should you go and sit with them and tell them about your day just for the hell of it, in case they can hear you, or should you leave them alone? I always felt that I was either intruding or ignoring them.'

There were two patients she did talk to and build up a rapport with in these last stages. When the first one of these died, she was very upset. 'I went to the office and was crying, and the other nurses were very supportive. It was all right – there was no sense that you should keep a stiff upper lip.'

With other patients she felt it would be almost an imposition to try and get through to them. 'In a lot of instances, you wanted to say: "It's OK, just go. Just go." You felt that they were clinging to life because they had to, or felt that they had to.' But she never did say that; it was too big a step for a patient's advocate to take. '*Could* you go in and say, "It's OK to die"? Is that immoral? Is that euthanasia?'

In the last week of the placement, at the end of July, the combined pressure of the ward, her own unresolved feelings about her friend's death and the impending separation from Mark took its toll. She had a panic attack in handover. Feeling dizzy and unable to catch her breath, she took herself off to the office and tried to calm down. But the symptoms wouldn't go and she was given two days' compassionate leave to rest and try and sort things out.

The placement ended with no further mishap, and Angela and Mark packed up the flat and prepared to move out. Before Mark left, they went on holiday together in France: afterwards Angela described it wistfully, remembering how they had lain on the grass at night and looked up at the stars.

Then it was back to London, the final parting from Mark

and the move into what seemed an impossibly cramped room in Alexandra Hall. At least her next placement, on a 'heavy' medical ward at Alf's, promised two advantages: it was a one-minute walk from her room and it would keep her so busy she'd have little time to think.

DURING A WEEK of hot, humid weather, the nurses on Howard Ward said goodbye to Julie, the little girl who had been brought in having had a fit, when her mother had tried to strangle her. It was the second time she had left Alf's; earlier she had been transferred to a different hospital, as she had continued to have fits and needed intensive care and investigations. They had brought the fits under control and she had returned to Howard to be rehabilitated. Now she was leaving – not to rejoin her mother (who had been charged by the police and whose future was uncertain) but to go to a foster home.

When Julie had been admitted two months earlier, Kate had been shocked by her injuries and angry at her mother for inflicting them. As the story unfolded, however, she had come to feel sympathy for the young mother. 'Julie and her mum are very good friends, and the reason her mum strangled her was because they'd both been abused by her boyfriend: the mother had been physically and sexually abused and Julie had been physically abused. And the mother's only a young girl and she didn't know what to do. She was at her wits' end. She'd tried to go into one of those refuges and he'd found her and brought her home, on and off for three years. Julie talks about it; "He's not coming, is he?" "No, no, you're safe here." "He was a naughty boy." '

Julie's mother had been taken into custody when Julie was admitted. She was seen by a doctor who said she had no psychiatric problems, which meant that she had to be charged. She was released pending the court case and had access to Julie, coming to see her very regularly, but she was not able to take her home. The nurses did not know all the ins and outs of what had happened and the matter was now out of their hands.

Julie was not the only child at risk on Howard; there had been a spate of them recently, coming in with Child Protection Orders because of suspected abuse. Kate had noticed her own responses settling down into a pattern. "Initially you're always sickened and angry. Naturally you always care for children and their welfare, but then you just get to know the family and you get to know the child and it doesn't come into it any more. They become another patient who needs a little bit more support and a little bit more care.'

She had also noticed that for children with chronic illnesses, the usual physical boundaries became blurred. 'These children get so much physical contact – they're always having something shoved into a vein, and of course a lot of mothers tend to sleep on the beds with their children because there's nowhere else to sleep. They're so used to physical contact that I'm not sure if they know where the boundaries are.'

The ward tried to protect children from 'inappropriate' behaviour by keeping male and female bays, but the toddlers tended to be mixed in together, and one day a little girl rushed up to Kate saying, 'Come and stop them, Simon and Helen are kissing!' Thinking she meant that they were exchanging pecks on the cheek (Simon and Helen were seven and six years old), Kate explained that this was quite all right; she was overruled by the sister who saw Simon, his arm strapped up to a drip, writhing around on top of Helen in the middle of the ward, with all the parents looking on.

'I took this little girl to one side and said, it's fine for you to play with Simon and to go into the Wendy House, but your body is yours and his body is his, and you can hold hands but you should be careful. If you don't feel comfortable, you should say no. And if he doesn't feel comfortable, he can say no too. She said, "He wasn't hurting me," and I said "No, but it isn't quite fair for him to lie on top of you" . . . it was very difficult, but I think she registered because afterwards he said, "Shall we go into the Wendy House?" and she said, "I think I'm going to say no." '

Kate was now completely at home on Howard, and was fairly well-acquainted with Walsh, the children's oncology ward downstairs. At weekends, many of the patients on both wards went home, and a slimmed down contingent of nurses would usually move the remaining children on Howard down to Walsh, and do their shifts down there. It meant that the hospital saved money on nurses and Howard meanwhile got a thorough clean and tidy up.

It was a good arrangement from Kate's point of view, as it gave her many weekends off. When it was her turn to go down to Walsh, however, she found it a strain. The nursing was more specialized, revolving around the children's chemotherapy: much checking of IV apparatus, taking observations, changing dressings and training parents to be able do these same tasks at home. Moreover, there were power struggles between the sisters of the two wards, which meant that nurses did not always have all the information they needed on one another's patients.

'There's not much difficulty from the junior staff level, but at the senior level they're fiercely protective of their children and their illnesses. You tend to get really poor handover: it should be really detailed with the name and age of the child and what treatment they're getting, but instead they'll just say, for example: "Annie: her temperature's up this morning." And you're wondering, what's the matter with her then? You haven't a clue who she is, what bed she's in, how old she is. So you say, "But I don't know the patient," and they say, "Oh, but you don't need to know the diagnosis." '

Matters came to a head one Saturday when Kate and one sister from Howard moved their patients down on to Walsh and were told that the handover between Walsh shifts had started without them and was now nearly finished. They had to give the information about their own patients without receiving any in return and a little while later the regular Walsh staff went to tea break together, leaving Kate and her sister with all the patients.

'There was this girl in a side ward and her Imed was bleeding, so I went into her room and was trying to work out her drip and after about five minutes she said to me: "Why aren't you wearing a pink gown?" And I looked at her and said, "Sorry?" And she said: "I've just had total body irradiation. You're highly infectious to me at the moment [radiation reduces patients' natural immunity] and you're supposed to be wearing a pink gown and gloves and all that sort of business." It was like – oh my *God*! But if she'd been properly handed over, or there had been a notice on the door, I would have known.

'Luckily I didn't touch her or breathe over her. I had my back to her and was working on the machine. But when I said to the sister that I had done it, we had to fill out an official form. My sister did shout at the other sisters who were supposed to be on duty – right in the middle of the ward. Eventually we had handover at about seven o'clock at night when there were only about two hours to go. It's stupid but it is a power struggle between the two wards. At least now, I think the senior nurse is looking into the whole thing.'

Kate was now beginning to detach herself emotionally from Howard and from Alf's. The house that she and Paul were having built was nearly finished and arrangements for the September wedding were well advanced. She would be leaving in August, with two weeks to spare, and she was now regularly reading the nursing magazines for job advertisements. She was also listed as an occasional employee of the health authority in south Shropshire, so she was able to apply for internal vacancies there. She was currently applying for a part-time post as outpatients' nurse at a cottage hospital near her home. It would mean running a number of clinics and seeing many patients without much continuity. She wasn't sure she wanted it, but jobs were scarce and choice was a luxury she couldn't afford.

Nor could anyone else. The precariousness of Alf's position was brought home to all the nurses when they received letters with their pay cheques asking if they would like to take early retirement or redundancy. It was a clear signal to everyone that in future they would have to fight to keep their jobs.

Reluctantly, some nurses were starting to leave, deciding that they had better pre-empt the rush. It was not a popular thing to do, but Kate could see no alternative for any of them. 'One of the nice sisters here has just left and people gave her a bit of stick, but in a few months' time everyone's going to be looking for G grade posts. There's all this talk of setting up a network whereby you have to employ London nurses over anyone else. That would be actively discriminating against other nurses in the country because there's going to be such a surplus of London nurses. But in a few years' time the problem will be nationwide anyway – all the inner cities are going to lose their hospitals.'

Although Kate had always planned to leave Alf's in the summer and get a job in the country, she was still haunted by what the closures would mean for staff and patients: 'I had a terrible dream. I dreamed that it was a Monday and the hospital was going to close on the Wednesday and I was thinking, how can we move these people? How can we physically move all these people with bits and things in them, here and there? They're not ready to go. Do we just close the doors and hand in our uniforms and let the patients get themselves out if they can . . .?'

*

RACHEL ALSO spent July and August on Howard. At long last the child branch rostered service had begun and she enjoyed the continuity of ten whole weeks on the ward. As she had hoped, the placement gave her a chance to consolidate the skills she had learnt there in spring. She was lucky in seeing a wide variety of patients – everything from tonsilectomies to children recovering from traffic accidents, from bowel disease to children having their ears pinned back. As she was now a full member of the nursing staff, Rachel did night shifts and weekends (though she never went down to Walsh, as it was decided the students wouldn't know enough about the specialized care to be a help) and was assigned special patients.

One of these was a girl with a new stoma, whom Rachel cared for immediately after her operation. 'On the first day she was really quiet; she was in pain and wasn't really with it. The second day you could tell there was that psychology of the altered body coming in. She didn't want to look at it and she didn't want to bend in the middle – she was really rigid. She had to get out of bed and she didn't want to. She was totally terrified and I kept on saying, "She's not talking and it's really bothering her, maybe someone should talk to her." And I went in the third day and she was in floods of tears about how she was going to be different, because no one else at school had one of these. She had a really big cry, "Why me?" and all the rest, and then in the afternoon she was terrific. It was almost as though she'd decided: right, this is it and I've got to get on with it. She was much better after that. It was really good to see and a real buzz for me.'

Meanwhile, Rachel was awaiting the results of the exam she had taken in June. The child branch students had longer to wait than the others, thanks to an administrative hitch ('Apparently one of the markers forgot to mark them, can you believe it?') and all the set became jumpy. Rachel needn't have worried, however: she passed well.

There were other things going on in Rachel's life besides work. She was due to be a bridesmaid at her sister's wedding in August, and was making fairly frequent trips home to be fitted for the dress, shoes and so on. ('I keep having visions of leaving the shoes half way down the aisle and falling over and ending up with the dress over my head.') In the middle of the preparations, her other sister announced her engagement, set a wedding date for the following year and promptly booked Rachel as bridesmaid again. At the end of July she and three of her colleagues from the branch decided that they'd had enough of the nurses' home and moved into a shared flat above an off licence, a couple of miles north of Alf's. And she and her boyfriend Robbie agreed to call it a day.

When she called me to give me her new address, Rachel was half excited, half tearful. She and Robbie had been together a long time and the break would be a big change. It was amicable however, so amicable that he soon came down to stay a weekend in the flat. He then planned another visit, and Rachel wasn't sure if quite so much contact was what she'd had in mind.

In the event, Rachel's placement on Howard ended in a flurry of pre-wedding activity. The wedding itself was a success, the party lasted well into the night and Rachel sat up through the dawn swallowing Alka-Seltzer and writing a project which had somehow fallen by the wayside and had to be in on Monday. She thought at the time that she was doing it rather well. Several weeks later she was flabbergasted to discover that the markers thought so too: she got 70 per cent on it, her best mark yet.

On HAMILTON WARD the summer months were proving rewarding for Christine, too. In June her reminiscence group came into being: representatives of Age Concern and a local initiative called Age Exchange came to St Wenceslas to lead the first of five nurse-and-client sessions. Four wards were taking part and two clients came from each. The idea was that the same clients would come to each meeting, get to know one another and grow used to talking about their memories.

It would be a gradual process: one of the characteristics shared by most elderly and confused people in St Wenceslas is that they are reluctant to do anything new. It requires so much effort, mental and physical, and it feels dangerous. Most of the clients at the first meeting had been persuaded to come and needed constant encouragement from the nurses.

There was a nurse for each client. Two of these nurses – Christine and another – would be permanent members of the group and would eventually pass on the skills they had learnt to other colleagues. Perhaps inevitably, given St Wenceslas' tight budget, the other nurses were made up of agency and part-time staff who might or might not be available to attend the next meeting.

Christine's client was Grace. Over the past weeks she had managed to get Grace to open up with her in private chats and she thought the group might encourage her to take more part in the life of the ward.

The 'trainers' from Age Concern and Age Exchange had brought along a variety of aids and they began the session by getting group members to throw a ball from one to another, saying their name as they caught it. This went on for ten minutes to help orientate the clients.

The group then split into nurse – client pairs and everyone chose something from a big bag of household objects and talked to his or her partner about it. The nurses' role was to give a lead and then encourage the clients to talk.

Grace chose a jelly mould. She told Christine that they'd had one like it in her family home and that when she was young she had helped her mother make jelly once a week. Then she talked a little about her parents.

After this, everyone got back into the general group, the

nurses contributed their memories and encouraged their clients to do the same. It was slow going but most people were able to say something.

Christine later identified the main part of the nurse's role as listening to the client. Although she didn't analyse the skills involved (that's not the way she talks), her account of it put me in mind of Nicola's observations on the awareness group at the Link and John's skill in drawing people out. Christine described how looking at a photograph of a street market would get the clients talking about what food they used to eat and where they used to buy it, and what struck me was how fluid and communal this process of memory-by-association was. The nurses need to be alert to the currents of memory in the disjointed talk, and help the clients draw their memories from it.

(I must admit that I squirmed when I first heard about using plastic fruit and pictures to prompt memories: it sounded so patronizing. Now I realized that on the contrary, it is a way of standing back and appealing to the clients' senses directly, igniting their memories with the minimum of interference.)

The good effects of the group were apparent in several of the clients, including Grace. Christine noticed it after the second session. Grace hadn't wanted to come to this; just like on the first occasion, she had to be persuaded to attend. But once in the session she responded well, remembering some of the others from the previous time, and when she went back to Hamilton she talked to some of her neighbours, telling them what had happened.

As the sessions continued, every fortnight, the trainers led the group on to more active pursuits. Instead of just talking about random items, they took themes: they began to 'make a market', using objects and pictures cut out of magazines. They made a collage of the seaside. At each stage of these activities, the nurses asked questions and encouraged the clients to exchange memories, and details of the clients' young lives gradually built up.

'Grace told us that she used to buy meat from the butcher, but he used to come to the house, she didn't go to the shop. And she never bought fish. Now we know why she doesn't like it, she's not used to it. When we made the collage of the seaside, she remembered that she used to work in a café.'

After each session (which lasted one hour), Christine would report back to the other nurses on Hamilton and tell them what had happened in the group. It was a kind of handover. She wanted to interest more nurses in reminiscence therapy and was hoping that once she had learnt the skills needed, she would be able to train several of her colleagues. The interest was polite but not overwhelming. Still, it was evident that the clients were benefiting from the group and the trainers from Age Concern and Age Exchange were keen; indeed, after the initial five sessions were finished, they wanted to continue coming. But Christine felt that it was important for the nurses to take over now, so the trainers withdrew and the group divided up according to wards, the idea being that the 'trained' nurses would pass on their skills to colleagues and more clients could become involved.

Reminiscence therapy was not the only involvement of the charities with the wards: Age Concern also helped organize several outings for clients, providing transport to take them to parks and gardens and on one occasion to a concert. It made a big difference to the ward now that there was transport available and three of Christine's patients went outside on one trip or another. Mary, the frail lady who had worn the pink dressing gown, went to a park. She also went to chapel in the hospital every week, as she liked to sing. Sally, a new patient and a music lover, went to the concert. Grace was finally persuaded that she should go on one of the park trips, even though Christine couldn't accompany her. (She came back reporting that she had enjoyed it.) And when Edie went as one of a group to a nearby shopping centre – an outing Christine did go on – she was exhilarated and came back to the ward saying that she'd been taken to Spain.

It was a much happier time than the winter had been. All Christine's clients were doing well and only one person on the whole ward had died since May. Her relations with her colleagues were better too. There was still the odd grumble at her eagerness to promote what some saw as extra work, but it was generally good natured. Besides, now that hospital management was insisting on regular ward audits, it was useful to have Christine to do all the standard setting, to oversee the implementation of the goals and to liaise with the people from the 'Validation Group' at Alf's, who came visiting to see what had been achieved (though some of the nurses still seemed inclined to think she was doing this for her own amusement).

Christine also received a small piece of official recognition for the memorial service she had organized on the ward in the spring. She reported on it briefly to a meeting of nurses, presided over by Alf's Chief Nurse, Miss Miller, who had been impressed and commended the initiative. On the career development front, Christine was still wary of doing a full-time conversion course, but was looking forward to the specialist course on care of the elderly which she would be starting in October. The course would bring her up to date with some of the latest developments in elderly care and earn her a sizeable number of points towards a diploma-level qualification, should she decide to do the conversion course. Her husband had made no demur when she told him about it.

Life at home was busy. Her sister and her family came to England for a holiday and stayed with her throughout August. There was much meeting up of family members and sightseeing. Christine saw them when she was off duty (and when this coincided with their times in) and in the second half of August she took two weeks leave so that she could spend some leisurely time with them.

During the summer the question of the new nursing home, the relocation of clients and the redeployment of staff had been floating round as ever. It seemed neither more nor less urgent than before and Christine was resigned to an indefinite period of inaction. However, while she was away one of her colleagues phoned to tell her that the acting nurse manager of continuing care had called a meeting of the enrolled nurses on Hamilton to discuss their future. In a nutshell, there was none: the nursing home would be employing RGNs and support workers, but there would be no enrolled nurse posts. Instead, for Christine and her fellows there would be 'options'.

This put something of a dampener on the end of her leave. When she arrived back on the ward, anxious to hear about these options, the other enrolled nurses were off duty, so she had to go to Personnel. Her options turned out to be: doing the two-year conversion course to become an RGN; doing a six-week course to become a support worker, or redundancy. If she did the conversion course, there was no guarantee of a job at the end of it. If she became a support worker she would almost certainly be re-employed, in a position with much less responsibility and much lower pay. Initially she would continue to be paid at her current rate, but management could not say for how long; afterwards her salary would drop and so would her pension entitlement. Stunned, Christine asked about redundancy. Given her length of service, she was told, early retirement might be the better option. She requested some facts and figures on both and was promised that they would be sent to her home. She was asked if she could make her decision swiftly – say, within a week.

That was Wednesday; on Saturday morning the calculations arrived at her house. It was a peculiar weekend. Christine discussed the options with her husband, her son and her daughter. The amount of time and effort involved in a conversion course had always been a stumbling block, even when it had seemed a good bet in career terms; now it looked like a lot of work for no security at all. She might well end up registered but unemployed. Conversely, if she became a support worker she would be accepting demotion. She would have to stop using the skills and experience of twenty-five years' nursing and spend the rest of her career making beds and serving meals, for a paltry wage. Oddly enough, this did not attract.

So within a few hours, it became inevitable that she would leave. She studied the figures: of the two packages on offer, early retirement was definitely the better. That, therefore, was the one she would take.

When she returned to St Wenceslas the next week, Christine made an appointment with Jack Williams (the person now acting as Senior Nursing Officer at St Wenceslas) and gave him her decision. They agreed on the end of October as the date for her to go. Under the terms of the pension scheme, she could continue working part-time afterwards, and it was settled that she would immediately return to Hamilton for one or two days a week as an agency nurse. She would 'of course' be employed at a lower grade than previously and for less money.

It had all happened extraordinarily quickly: within seven days Christine had gone from being someone who was experienced and valued within the NHS and deeply involved in improving its nursing care, to being someone who had no place in it. When she told me what had happened (on the telephone), she refused to comment on it at all beyond saying that it was strange and laughing a little. At the time, I was sure she must be angry and hurt, and hiding it; now I think that perhaps she was simply stunned.

One thing which worried her in the short term was our working together, now that her status was changing; she asked me to check with Jack Williams that it would still be all right for her to take part in this book. (All the way through, she has been assiduous about getting the hospital's permission for every form of contact with me.) I made the call reluctantly, feeling that instead of asking dispensation on Christine's behalf I should be berating this man and all of St Wencelas' management and pointing out its disloyalty, stupidity and wilful waste of human resources. However, there was no need: within thirty seconds it was evident that Jack Williams felt much the same way.

'We have had changes thrust on us from above,' he said bitterly. He was very sorry that Christine had come to her 'quite understandable' decision. He had been very sorry to see his predecessor, Mrs Aballa, go. In fact, I got the impression that he was sorry about everything, not least that he was here, having to implement policies he abhorred.

Poor Jack Williams: his is the recurring dilemma for nursing and medical managers in the 1990s NHS. Should they leave, when asked to implement policies with which they violently disagree? Or should they stay, and try to influence or at least mitigate in some small way? It is an interesting moral question. And then of course, they too have jobs to look after – if they leave this one, will they ever get another?

But it was academic to Christine now. Whatever happened in the loftier reaches of St Alphege's Trust, she would be going at the end of October. Grace, Edie and Mary, the rehabilitation group, the individual performance reviews and the ward audits would just have to get along without her.

Autumn

SEPTEMBER CAME to the Link and, with the arrival of the new month, the end of Catherine's first programme was in sight. She was feeling very much better about it. Many of her doubts and frustrations had faded – imperceptibly to her, strikingly to me. The big change was the confidence she had acquired in running groups.

'I actually enjoy doing the groups and I've had a fair amount of positive feedback as well, which is nice. People think I'm an expert on relaxation which makes me die with laughter! Apparently I've *cured* people! I read to them from scripts; it's not guided fantasy ("You are lying on a beach...") but physiological: "Relax your right arm..." I think people like my voice. I've done a tape at the audio-visual department and people think that's wonderful! But I'm literally doing the work the night or morning before. I did a theory group this afternoon (Nicola helps me with it now) and the group was at one and we were discussing it at twelve. I feel confident enough to do that now; I feel I can get myself out of jams.'

The time management group had also been a success. Although it had gained only one more member, the work they were doing was well suited to a small group. Two of the three clients made real progress, achieving the goals they had set for themselves and doing more and more constructive things with their time as the weeks went on.

The third member, Nicola's favourite client Victor, was hampered by his very high anxiety levels. 'He's so terribly, terribly anxious and concerned that we're going to be upset or disappointed in him. He finds it difficult to plan in advance, it goes against the grain with him. But he says it does make him think about what he's going to do at the weekend and things like that. That's very important as he lives on his own in a little bedsit and it can be very lonely for him.'

Although Victor wasn't yet making strides in time management, he was enjoying the group so much that he asked if he could do it again. The answer was very likely to be yes, as the Link evidently suited him. 'He's been so isolated and now, in a way, he's blossoming.'

On the whole, Catherine preferred the more structured groups. She enjoyed taking assertiveness with Helen, but found the women's group, also with Helen, hard going. 'It's never really taken off because the members find it quite difficult to express their feelings. A lot of that is because they feel they would be dumping on the other people in the group – they're very, very careful not to do that. The group goes for a little while then stops and you have to kick start it again. But it *is* beginning to work and I think some of them will go back into it on the next programme.'

Given a free choice, Catherine would have liked to take more structured groups. But she had come to realize that certain nurses seemed to 'own' certain groups. 'Helen seems to own assertiveness and stress management. John does the psychodynamic groups like drama therapy and awareness. Roberta does the low-key groups.' And as Catherine was already doing relaxation on her own and time management with Roberta, besides the groups she shared with Helen, there was not much room for her to extend her range in the short term. 'In any case, if I'm going to have ten clients on the next programme, I'll have more to do with them.'

Catherine was still having some problems with her new job. The main one was adjusting to the very structured way of working which prevailed at the Link: knowing what she would be doing every day of the week made her feel claustrophobic. The nine-to-five hours, which she had expected to be such a bonus, also proved problematic: her partner Bob was still working predominantly late shifts, so she saw very little of him. Too often, she spent the evenings at home, alone or pottering round with her flatmate, feeling cooped up.

However, the severe doubts and anxieties of the early weeks were gone now. She had settled with herself that she would definitely stay at the Link at least six months, and she even turned down an invitation to apply for the post of community nurse attached to Wilcox, her old ward. Instead, her job-hunting energies were being deployed for Bob, who was looking for community-based posts as well. 'And we're trying to organize a holiday. We think we can get time off together in a few weeks' time, so we're just going to go abroad somewhere, wherever we can find, before they stop us!'

For NICOLA, September brought the prospect of a move out of the Link, and exams. She had not been able to postpone sitting the exams, so she was working hard to catch up on her studies. Happily, her father seemed to be getting better, or at least stabilizing, and she felt less worried about him. As she began disengaging herself from close contact with clients at the Link, Nicola let the staff know that she would be very interested in a post there when she registered.

'The amount you can learn there is so good and the supervision is so good and they're the type of clients I like working with. This is very much the "soft" end of psychiatry. I think the acute wards are the psychiatric equivalent of working in A & E: you need to be always on your toes, assessing situations, you get the adrenalin rush every now and then. But it's not for me. I enjoy the education side of working at the Link and I like the fact that you're giving people something that they can take away and use.'

She liked the people at the Link too. They formed an easygoing unit and sometimes went out together socially. Nicola had become part of that over the summer. In early September, Helen got married and Nicola went to the wedding with the other Link staff; the next day, which was a warm, sunny Sunday, she spent with David, her partner, and Catherine. (Bob was working, as usual.)

Nicola was now looking forward to the end of the course. She was twenty-eight and felt it was time that her life expanded to contain more than work, placements and exams. She was also longing to be paid a decent salary. 'David's a solicitor so he's quite well paid and I can never afford to do the things he'd like us to do. I want to pay my way, I wouldn't like to take David's money, and I've managed on the bursary so far, by being careful. But it would be nice not to have to be so careful!'

Meanwhile, she was busy drawing up plans for her next placement which was officially her elective. The students on the mental health branch had a reasonably free hand, within limits: they had to work within the St Alphege's and Wavetree Health Authority and Nicola had to go to an institution as she had just come from the community.

As she reviewed the places where she had worked and sought ideas for new places she might try, one institution kept coming back into her mind: the Grange, up in the north of Wavetree borough, where she had worked a year ago. Her time there had been mixed and interesting. As a private hospital, it had shown her a very different environment from those she had grown used to since; she began to think seriously about returning for a second look.

OVER ON MARLOWE, meanwhile, Liz Howlett had her hands full. It had been a busy summer and the nurses were being asked to work harder for less reward. The new ward had been put on hold and an atmosphere of uncertainty had crept into Marlowe. There had been wranglings over nurses' time off.

'Andrew, our senior nurse, has told us that if we claim back time off we're owed for working weekends, we should shorten the hours we're claiming to reflect the higher rate of pay we've got for those shifts.'

The nurses were very unhappy about it: they argued that they didn't usually choose to work weekends, but were asked to, and that the unsocial hours supplement they received was a compensation for losing time with friends and family. Days off in lieu, which usually took place during the week, did not restore that to them. The matter was stirring a good deal of resentment and some of the nurses were inclined to answer the hospital in kind.

'One of the other sisters has said that the next time she's asked to stay late, she'll say no. But no isn't in my vocabulary. A lot of the nice feeling about being part of an organic team has gone from the NHS since the hospitals became trusts and everyone's watching their backs and their jobs. I still let nurses go early after a hard shift, but I feel a twinge each time I do. On this issue, I can see both the staff's and Andrew's point of view. I wouldn't want to be a manager.'

Liz hadn't gone abroad this summer, as she usually did, because she was in the process of buying out her flatmate and she needed to save money. Instead she had gone to visit a friend in Yorkshire for a week and spent a second week off at home, decorating. Having decided that she wanted to live alone, after years of amicable sharing, she was now impatient to take sole possession. Her friend had been due to move out in August, but had suffered a series of hitches with her new place, and so in early September, Liz was still sharing her home. Fond of her friend as she was, she was beginning to chafe at the delay.

As summer gave way to autumn, there were some good

developments on Marlowe. One was the establishment of a formal link with Natalie, one of the liaison psychiatrists who worked with patients on Alf's non-psychiatric wards. 'She's been coming over several times a week, giving us general support and asking us what our concerns are, how we'd like her to work with the patients. Now we've established a regular meeting when the nurses get together with her and review the patients. If we think a particular patient needs help, Natalie will go along informally and introduce herself, see if they want to talk.' Sometimes the contact would remain casual; in other cases, a patient might be officially referred for psychiatric treatment.

'Quite a few people are being referred on now. We've always known that a lot of people needed to see a psychiatrist or a psychologist, but when we used to refer them before, unless you get someone who's well-versed in AIDS, they're reluctant to treat patients unless you can actually diagnose an organic cause for things. Natalie's good because she's willing to address the problems, whether they have an organic origin or not.'

The other good development was over the heads of the ward staff: hospital management called a special meeting for doctors and nurses in the AIDS department and passed on some good news. Word had come (discreetly) from the region that A & E was to get a reprieve. It would not be closing for a few years yet and therefore support services in the rest of the hospital would continue to run, in the medium term at least. Building on the new AIDS and immunology ward would now be going ahead, as quickly as possible.

It was very cheering news. Optimism had held up pretty well on Marlowe, despite the odd tremor, and now the staff felt vindicated. 'The general feeling now is that it will take more than a few ministers messing up to see the end of us.'

All was not harmonious on the ward, however. There was tension building up between Mark, one of the staff nurses, and Rowena, a doctor. It was nothing very important: just that Mark had questioned Rowena a few times on her approach to treating a particular patient and Rowena was not someone who liked being challenged, particularly by nurses. Rowena had begun to be noticeably cool towards Mark.

There had been problems with doctor–nurse relations before. Early in the summer a Somalian woman, Diole, had been admitted with a chest infection, and when she began behaving strangely, Liz had suspected a brain tumour. 'She was unsteady on her feet and she used to sit on the loo for hours – sometimes she'd spend all night in the bathroom. There were numerous family and friends and one of them, a British man, said it was a cultural thing. She liked the bathroom because it was cooler. She liked to run the water because it reminded her of home.'

Liz wasn't convinced. 'I know from some of the other African people we've had, they often grieve when they're sick. They *don't* like too much interference, they're very private. But these other things didn't add up, and it's very easy to say, "Oh well, it's because she's from another country." '

She raised the matter with Jean, one of the two senior house officers attached to the ward, but got the same response. 'Jean's worked abroad a lot, and I was getting messages back from her via the nurses: "Oh, Jean says it's cultural. Jean says this is how they cope when they're not well. Jean says we don't understand Africans." Well, maybe I don't understand Africans but I know they don't just not bother to go to the toilet because they're sick, and I know they don't spend all night with their head on the floor.'

When Diole started vomiting, the doctors sent her for a scan. Sure enough, she had a brain tumour. Liz was stung that her observations had been written off as culturally biased: she considered herself more sensitive than many people to the rights and needs of African HIV patients. She was also exasperated at the way her fellow nurses appeared to have been steamrollered by a doctor's opinion.

'Jean's a good doctor and a nice woman and I like her, but she can be quite snappy and I know that when she said what she did to the nurses, they wouldn't have questioned it. They'd just have gone away. I did ask her about it and she said, "I wish people would stop saying I said it was cultural, because I didn't." I think actually she did, but she probably didn't mean it was *all* cultural.'

In any event, Liz had put the disagreement down, somewhat wryly, to experience. No harm had come to the patient from it: unfortunately, Diole's condition was inoperable and wouldn't have been affected by earlier screening. And she felt that perhaps she would be listened to more attentively next time. She hoped that the needling between Mark and Rowena would blow over in the same way, but she had her doubts.

The biggest shadow over the ward at the moment was the situation of two of the patients. Tim and Louis were both very ill and both enmeshed in complications, Tim's personal, Louis's medical.

Tim had been ill for about a year. Just before Christmas he had come in, been diagnosed with a cerebral tumour and received chemotherapy. He'd done very well and had returned home. He lived alone but his partner of eight years, Roy, spent a good deal of time with him and helped to look after him. During the first half of the year Tim had come back into Marlowe a few times for drug therapy; when he'd come in earlier this summer, it was apparent to the staff that he was going downhill. He couldn't talk very well; he was incontinent and his mental state had deteriorated so that although he was rational and knew what was going on, he was vague. His parents had visited him several times on that stay, and had decided to come up from their home in the country and move in with him when he went home again.

Liz had her doubts at the time: she knew that Roy was used to looking after Tim and wondered how he and Tim's parents would cope with one another. Unfortunately, the answer was not very well. The parents and Roy kept in touch with the hospital separately, asking the staff's advice on how to look after Tim and what he could or couldn't do, so the staff received a picture (mainly through Roy) of what was happening in the flat. It seemed that Tim's parents were unwilling to acknowledge the depth of Roy's relationship with their son and Roy, who had been planning to go on caring for his partner, felt pushed out.

'There's some suspicion among the nurses that the parents have put pressure on Tim, said things like, "Oh, Roy will never be able to look after you." Out of concern for Tim, but on another level, they're taking him away from him. For instance, Tim was going to go and spend the weekend with Roy, at his flat, but I think he was discouraged.'

Roy continued to go and see Tim but would often feel so unwelcome that he had to leave. He was bitterly hurt by it and in the last week of July he went to stay with friends in France.

At the end of the week, Tim's parents brought him in to Marlowe. He was very ill indeed and unable to communicate. The doctors said there was nothing they could do for him and the staff expected him to die quickly, within a few days. Roy had been calling in from France to ask after Tim and he now called the nurses to ask what the outlook was and whether they thought he should come home. As Tim couldn't speak and no one really knew how much he could understand, the nurses couldn't ask him what he wanted. Roy himself was torn about whether or not he should come. 'He didn't know if he could face the parents' coolness and their neglect of his relationship with Tim. He was so hurt by it.'

Initially, Roy didn't come back. But Tim rallied over the weekend, though he was still unable to communicate, and next time Roy called and heard this, he decided to come home. He was due back on Monday.

I saw Liz that afternoon, and she was nervous on his

behalf: 'He's coming in to see Tim this evening. I think he'll probably arrange it for a time the parents aren't there, but he doesn't argue with them anyway; he just leaves if he gets frustrated.'

Liz felt the strain of trying to mediate between Roy and Tim's parents; and the fact that the breach remained largely unacknowledged – or at least unspoken – only made it harder. She was also terribly sad for them all: in their different ways they were each in such pain and in the middle of it all, Tim was dying.

Louis was also probably dying – at least, that was what the doctors at Alf's thought. The trouble was that no one really knew what was the matter with him: they knew he had HIV and some kind of brain infection; they knew he had been treated in a hospital in Sussex and then sent to a rehabilitation unit. But no one had been able to diagnose what he was suffering from and therefore no one could be sure of the right treatment. Nor could they give him a prognosis.

Louis was very badly disabled when he was admitted. His speech was slurred; he couldn't stand and he couldn't move his left arm. He could hold a short conversation, though it cost him a painful effort of concentration, and Liz wasn't sure how many things he could hold in his mind at once.

He got a bit better while he was on Marlowe and the doctors talked to him about his options. The main thrust of their message was that they didn't know what was wrong with him, and thought that the likelihood was that he wouldn't recover. But they weren't sure and so he had to choose whether to continue receiving palliative care and hope for the best, or to go on and have a biopsy so that they could run further diagnostic tests. If they came up with a firm diagnosis, they might be able to increase his remaining time through treatment. But he should be aware that the biopsy carried a risk: he would need a general anaesthetic which always had a risk factor, probably a greater one for someone in his weakened state; and there was a chance that the biopsy might make him worse.

Louis decided to go for the biopsy. But he was very disoriented and kept asking the nurses what they thought his chances were; as no one could give a confident answer, they found it very upsetting. 'There's diagreement among the nursing staff. Some nurses feel he's too disabled to get any benefit from it. To some extent, that's true, but Louis wants it so I feel that the nurses must be brought round to see that although they believe he shouldn't go through it, they can't impose their moral beliefs on him. One or two nurses feel that the doctors weren't completely honest in the way they presented his options, but they were, because I was there when they did it. And then some people feel that he's not mentally clear enough to make the decision – but I think that's a terrible assumption to make.'

The nurses talked about it amongst themselves, and although everyone agreed that all was being done with Louis's best interests at heart, some of Liz's colleagues were still unhappy about it.

Louis's mother and sister were also unhappy. At different stages they had been told different things about his illness and by the time he came to Alf's, none of them knew any longer what to expect.

'The trouble is, he's been given mixed messages. One lot has talked about rehabilitation, you might get better, think positive. Then this medical opinion comes along and says, "Well, we don't know what's wrong with you, so it doesn't look as if you're going to get better." It's not fair on him. He said, "If someone could tell me something definite, a time: six months, or till Christmas, I'd be happy with that." '

In the same week that Louis went for biopsy and Tim was brought in speechless and dying, the resentment between Rowena and Mark came to a head. During a ward round, in front of Liz, the registrar and some students, Rowena implied to a patient that Mark's care wasn't reliable. The registrar immediately asked her what she meant and Rowena back-pedalled and ended up looking somewhat foolish – to Liz's grim satisfaction. But Liz was furious: 'It makes me so angry that someone would do that, insinuate that a nurse wasn't doing his or her job properly just to make themselves look superior. I spoke to her about it afterwards. I told her that wasn't the way to go about things and what with that and the registrar not letting her get away with it, I don't think she'll do it again in a hurry.'

Luckily for everyone, Rowena was due to move away from the ward almost immediately. She would be coming back to the hospital to take clinics but wouldn't return to Marlowe. Her replacement was a woman who had worked in an AIDS rehabilitation centre, so Liz had hopes of someone with a more positive attitude to nurses.

In the meantime, the events of the last week had left her feeling wrung out. All she wanted to do was take some time off and be alone in her flat. 'I can't wait to be living alone,' she said, with a tinge of desperation. 'To have no one but myself to think about.'

'THINGS ARE looking very, very good for A & E,' Janet said cheerfully, in her cubby-hole of an office. I had just been hearing as much from Liz on Marlowe, but now I got the full, unofficial story.

It seemed that the promised consultative period was coming up trumps for A & E. 'Basically, the region have now replied to their own consultation document – I don't really understand that bit! – and they have said that although they ultimately aim to close the A & E department at Alf's, they realize that they need to get support services up and running first. That means a larger A & E department at the Wavetree end, with a hospital able to take the extra patients that are coming through. Which means doubling the size of the Wavetree. They also acknowledge that they'll need better community resources for the patients – the GPs will have to provide a better service. Until these things happen, they would not envisage closing Alf's. Now for that, we could be looking at anything between five to ten years. The capital investment needed at the Wavetree,' she added happily, 'is in excess of 20 million.'

Janet's view was that nothing would change drastically within the next five years. It was an outlook shared by other departments too: the construction of the new AIDS and immunology ward seemed to offer concrete proof that the threat was receding.

It made a big difference to morale. Although from the outside the department looked as embattled as ever – a full waiting area, '$2\frac{1}{2}$ hours' written up on the board that indicated maximum waiting times, handwritten posters urging people to sign petitions and write to their MPs – through the swing doors the atmosphere was discernibly lighter. They were short-staffed and Janet was exhausted after having worked several six-day weeks in a row, sometimes doing double shifts in order to fulfil her site duty, but at least A & E appeared to have a future.

The management aspect of Janet's work was very much to the fore in September: when I saw her she was preoccupied with staffing and finance difficulties. For some time now, she said, she had been 'down two G grades and half an F grade' – in other words, the department was operating without one of its part-time and two of its full-time sisters. They had all gone on maternity leave; two were expected back, the third had just officially resigned to become a practice nurse. Recruiting her replacement would be a tortuous process, requiring lots of clearance from various bodies. Meanwhile, though absences could be covered by agency nurses, it wasn't the same as having experienced and committed senior staff.

And of course, it was more money out of the budget as each nurse on maternity leave receives a percentage of her salary.

'I have to say, maternity leave is crippling the NHS at the moment. Through every speciality, everyone is getting pregnant. It's not just us, I believe it's nationwide. It's all the people reaching the age where they feel they should now start a family or it will be too late.'

This is the kind of issue which, increasingly, exercises senior nurses in the NHS. Janet was quick to say that she supported women's rights to maternity leave and maternity pay; she thought cases of people being sacked for getting pregnant were appalling. But when experienced nurses took maternity leave, they left a skill vacuum behind them and she didn't think it was feasible for the NHS to go on dealing with it on an ad hoc basis. 'I think we'll have to devise a proper structured approach to maternity cover, especially where the person is going to be out for a year.'

Janet's own conditions of employment had changed recently. As part of a management review aimed at maximizing efficiency, senior A & E staff had recently been 'reassessed'. Janet had gone through an official interview in July and had immediately been confirmed in her job, keeping all the same responsibilities. However, her job title was changed. From now on she would not be called a Clinical Nurse Manager but a Senior Nurse and so she would be paid on a senior nurse scale – in other words less than before. Management had discovered a simple way of maximizing her efficiency! The cut was officially postponed as she had salary protection for a year; in practice she lost money immediately as she could no longer claim enhanced pay for working evenings and weekends.

At another time, she might have been angered by this. But now it just seemed part and parcel of working in a threatened area of the NHS, though she could have done without recurrent evenings and weekends on site duty. 'I've taken it up with the person who writes the rotas and told them that other people have got to start pulling their weight because there are some senior people in other departments who just don't do enough.'

Despite being so busy, Janet was in contemplative mood when we met. The season was changing and she was about to go away on holiday; perhaps she felt at one remove from the patients and the clinical work. She gave me the impression that she was trying to assess the way that A & E nursing was changing, and work out where she stood on matters of conscience and morality.

Throughout the year, the department had been treating a steady intake of drug overdoses and accidents. Some were deliberate suicide attempts; others were the result of recreational mishaps. The accident ODs tended to happen at weekends, when young people came in to the area for parties in warehouses and empty buildings. Ecstasy was the usual culprit: problems would arise not from direct overdoses, but from a combination of the drug, prolonged energetic dancing and badly ventilated surroundings leading to people becoming hot and dehydrated. If they had taken alcohol as well, the effects were worse.

'We had a sixteen-year-old who died a month ago. She had taken Ecstasy and become very dehydrated, very, very hot. Her friends had taken her outside and given her some orange juice. She'd become unconscious and inhaled it. Which is dreadfully sad because they had tried to do something about it. But the problem was still the drug – if she hadn't taken drugs she wouldn't have got into that state.'

As a nurse, it is not Janet's role to judge people. But as a nurse, her job also involves educating people about their health – and one woman's education is another person's unwarranted intrusion. In some cases, the patient doesn't even want to tell the staff about the drug.

'You can say to some, "I know you've taken Ecstasy," and

they say, "How?" "I can tell because your eyes are like saucers. The whites are just a rim, the pupils are like saucers." They say, "Well, I'm a safe user, a responsible user." But I say to them, "We had a sixteen-year-old dead last week and she thought she was responsible too. You cannot be responsible if you are taking something you do not know the consequence of."

'I always try and say that to them. All drugs are cut with other substances. People take things without knowing what's in them. Sometimes I say to them, "Why are you taking this crap? If I gave you a pile of salt, would you take that? You wouldn't touch it. Yet you take this and you don't know what's in it."

'They tend to be quite shocked. I think they don't expect you to do it, they expect you to be impartial. You're a nurse and you're not going to tell them off for doing something. But I see our role as a health educator as being much more than that.'

Whether patients took any notice of these ad hoc lectures (which were also quite forceful, if her sample to me was typical), Janet couldn't know. She felt it was part of her job to try and give them information, and point out that the choice was up to them. I suspected that it was also a fairly direct way of expressing her frustration at this self-inflicted harm; she agreed, but was adamant that she did it constructively, not to condemn.

More vexing, sometimes, was the question of deliberate overdoses. The drugs used were usually paracetemol and valium, and paracetemol in particular could have horrible consequences. Even if the patients were found alive and had their stomachs pumped, they could still die a few days later of liver failure. 'We've had a chap in here incredibly remorseful, but it's too late, you're into liver failure. The only thing you can do about it is a transplant.'

Again, there was an element of health education involved

here. Sometimes it had to be done against the clock: Janet had once had to persuade a teenage boy to accept the antidote to his paracetemol overdose while there was still time. 'I said, "It isn't a glamorous way to die. It's a long, slow painful death. It's not a TV programme, it's real life; we are talking *pain*. The choice is yours." '

By and large, Janet said, she did not get annoyed with people for inflicting damage on themselves in this way. 'You mean, "Stupid little cow, how could you do this? How could you do this to your mother?" ' No. Because I don't know what the situation is. What's presented to us is often a different side of the coin to what's presented to other people.

'My friend Mary was in hospital recently and said to me afterwards that she knew nurses weren't sympathetic to overdoses. I said, "I'm sorry but I don't think that's true." Some people are very desperate when they do this. Some people need a good ticking off because they've done it in a childish fit, to get back at somebody. And even then, though you can identify those people, you've got no right to do it, because you're not in their position. Mary said that a nurse on her ward had told everybody what this patient had done. That's very unprofessional. In fact, they could be disciplined because they are breaking confidentiality. It wasn't at this hospital, I hasten to add.'

Janet brooded for a while about this case and wished she had been in a position to do something about it. She was genuinely indignant about the unprofessionalism; the idea of such a lapse in standards evidently hurt her.

Listening to Janet asserting that she was 'generally very sympathetic' to attempted suicides, I thought of what Rachel had said about the nurses at the district hospital A & E, and their treatment of the young overdose patients: 'You almost felt like the staff were punishing them: "It's a horrible job, putting a tube down and pumping your stomach, and I really resent this because I don't want to do this and I don't enjoy this, and why were you so stupid?" '

I wondered now if this was fair. In a rushed A & E department, performing a procedure where time is of the essence, perhaps the nurses were simply concentrating on doing their job correctly. Perhaps also they were at a loss for what to say. After all, A & E culture is geared towards practical action; the nurses grow skilled at breaking bad news (and good), but they do not have much time to get to know patients, or a remit to give them psychological support in the way that, say, oncology nurses do.

Moreover, giving and receiving support depends on people being on each other's wavelength. Janet is an experienced senior sister who can find a response to most situations, but it was intriguing to speculate what Rachel would make of her 'sympathy'. Janet's style is straightforward and trenchant and in some circumstances it might be mistaken for callousness. If I were a patient, I think on the whole I'd appreciate her honesty. But then I'm thirty-five, not fifteen.

Certainly, when sympathy fails, honesty provides a good fall back. There was a habitual overdoser coming in frequently at the moment who, Janet acknowledged, strained her compassion. 'He actually said once, "I'm never going to do that again." I said, "Can I have that in writing please?" He said, "Do you want it in *blood*?" I said, "I think I'd better." Three days later he was in again with the same overdose. He's extremely manipulative and does it to get attention. He's well known to another hospital, who are treating him and know his problems. He's obviously got a need, he has a psychological problem, but the time and resources you have to put into this man actually do make me angry. He's in now – he has to have a huge amount of antidote given to him tomorrow. It ends up being very expensive in nursing time and hospital time, and you know he's going to do it again.'

Janet did not feel sympathy for this man, so did not try to express any. What she did owe him, she felt, was her professionalism and the comprehension which came from that. 'I let him know that I know why he's doing it – but not in a condemning way. I just say, "I'm aware of why you are doing this," like I might say to someone, "I know why you are shouting at me, it's because you're in pain." '

This, she felt, served two purposes: it laid down ground rules for the nurse–patient relationship and it siphoned off the emotion which might otherwise build up. 'I think you have to try and distance yourself from it and keep yourself in a purely nursing capacity, otherwise you get so wound up you can't get free. At the end of the day you have to say to people, "This is your choice." I'm a great one for telling people, "You have to choose. I'm not going to choose for you." A lot of people want you to choose for them, you know. They say to me, "Should I take time off work?" I say, "I don't know, I don't know how easy it is for you. You decide." '

At the moment, Janet had decided that she, at least, required some time off: two weeks, to be exact. 'I've gone through the whole summer without a break and it's too much. The last few weeks, I've been snapping at everyone, it's been like having PMT all the time. I haven't been able to do anything constructive about the problems that are around. I find that the only way to unwind is to go abroad and leave it all behind. I'm going to Crete now, and I'll be looking at some of the archaeological sites. That's my great interest. If ever I get to do a degree, I'd like to do it in archaeology.'

By the time Janet left for Crete, Kate Marshall had already said her more permanent goodbyes to Howard Ward and Alf's. September saw her in Shropshire. She'd felt some regret at leaving Howard, but none for London; she was quite ready to go home. Not that it was a peaceful homecoming. The wedding was three weeks away and although all the major preparations had been made, there was the inevitable, seemingly endless stream of small things to see to.

(It seems to be a law of nature that the longer in advance weddings are planned, the more last-minute rush they seem to involve.)

Many of the preparations were connected with Kate's parents' house, where the wedding was to be held. Kate's parents very sensibly took themselves off on holiday for the first two weeks of September, so they had a rest and she had the place to herself. She was able to unwind and get the last remnants of London out of her system, while checking the wedding arrangements and the progress of the brand new house which she and Paul would be moving into after their honeymoon.

This had been built on Paul's father's farm, chiefly a bull stud, with 150 bulls, a few pigs and other assorted farmyard creatures. The bulls were hired out for three months at a time and most of the year Paul's work centred round transporting them to the hiring farms. At the moment, however, the straw in the fields was ready for baling and Paul was working long hours at that.

The new house was built and semi-furnished, and would be ready for them to move into. The essentials were there: chairs, beds, a table, an Aga and a wood-burning stove. The rooms still lacked carpets but they could get round to those later. Ten days before the wedding, Kate's parents came home and the serious final preparations began. The weather turned temperamental, raining and shining in turns and making it impossible to predict what would happen on the day. One of the last things Kate did the night before was to make up a bed in the new house so that she and Paul would be able to go straight there when they arrived back from their honeymoon.

The next morning, the weather distinguished itself by being not only fine but warm and golden. Everything went well; eighty-eight guests enjoyed themselves without being rained on once, and Kate and Paul headed off to Sorrento for more sun.

When they came back, they settled in to the new house and Kate got some part-time nursing work. She usually worked three or four days every week, either at a tiny cottage hospital about ten miles away, or at a larger district general hospital, fifteen miles off. They were part of the same health authority and Kate had worked in both before. She knew staff (and sometimes patients) at each. At the district hospital in particular, there were nurses who had been at school with her and she enjoyed being back in their company.

At the cottage hospital, there were only sixteen beds, all for adults. The district hospital had the usual mix of medical, surgical, adults, children and elderly; there she began by working on a surgical ward.

'Things are done very differently up here. In Alf's, wherever you go there's a certain way of doing things and it's all more or less the same. Here, every ward has got its own way.

'On the surgical ward for instance, in the morning the senior staff nurse for the day takes over from the night staff while the rest of you go in and wash as many patients as you possibly can before 8 o'clock! Then at 8 o'clock you all sit down with the night shift and have handover. It takes about an hour because they all have a chat and a cup of tea. Then at 9 o'clock the real work starts, and you do that for about a quarter or half an hour, then they start letting you go off for your coffee break! It's very strange. Woe betide anyone who wants to go to the loo between eight and nine.'

This was very much old-fashioned nursing, with tasks being performed to a set routine. The patient-as-customer ethos prevalent in Alf's and other London hospitals had certainly not made much of a mark here. Kate found it all quite amusing, if slightly baffling, and was wary of rocking the boat. When she did now and then ask why things were done in a particular way, the answer was usually a mildly astonished stare and the phrase, 'Well, it's always been done like that.'

Similarly strange after life at Alf's was the way that people she scarcely knew recognized her. Paul's family were well known in the district and several times patients and staff were able to identify her, either by face or name, and informed her that she had recently got married. Mostly, she liked it – she'd had enough of big city anonymity – but it had its embarrassing side. 'A gentleman was in for a groin operation and I was sent in to shave him. Usually it's for a hernia, and you ask which side they're having done and shave that side. I asked this man and he said, "I'm having a vasectomy." So I went outside and asked the sister and she said, "You must shave everything."

'I went back in, and said, "Would you like to shave yourself?" He said, "No, no, I can't really see what's happening down there, I might cut myself. You do it." I was shaving him, asking him to move this and so on, it's a bit embarrassing, and I was chatting away trying to take our minds off it. I asked him what he did and he said, "I drive lorries" and before I thought, I asked if he knew Paul, because he spends so much time driving the bulls in lorries, and "Yes! Yes! Oh I know Paul . . ." it turned out he knew him really well. And there I was shaving him and trying desperately not to cut him. And the next day I saw him in the supermarket!'

One thing that was not such a change was the fact that both the district and the cottage hospital were under threat. The possibility of closure was recent news, and Kate found herself in the odd position of battle-hardened veteran, reassuring her new colleagues that the worst might not occur.

'They say, "How can you be so relaxed about it? You'll be out of a job too." But after going through it for all of the last year in London, I suppose I'm just used to it.'

Meanwhile, Kate was going ahead with her plan to apply for midwifery courses. In the long run, she thought, it was probably a very sensible career move: 'People will always have babies, even in the country.'

OCTOBER WENT swiftly for the enrolled nurses preparing to leave St Wenceslas. Christine made a conscious effort to untie herself from the sense of responsibility which she had always felt towards the ward as a whole. Once a part-timer, employed as an A grade (the same level at which the students were employed when they did agency work), she would not be able to go on being the ward manager's right-hand person. It wouldn't be feasible practically; it would not be fair on her fellow support workers for her to exceed her brief so dramatically; and she did not feel like doing it. In the past, her willingness to share the ward manager's burden had annoyed some of the other staff nurses; explaining to them that things would change was not without a certain grim pleasure.

'I said to them, "Up to the thirty-first of October, I'm willing to give you all the help you need. But after that don't come to me and ask me for help, because I won't know anything!"'

One week before leaving, she had mixed feelings about the impending change. She would miss the patients, she said, but she didn't expect to miss the staff. 'These people have hurt me so much at different times.'

I have had to employ narrator's privilege in writing about Christine's relations with her colleagues. In the chapters so far, when I have given glimpses of the problems she had experienced, I was drawing on information she had not yet given me in the interviews. She had hinted at a few difficulties and told me that the hospital management had specifically asked her to go to Hamilton to support the ward manager, but she had not gone further than that. It was only now that she was about to leave that she told me the story of the petty shoe-hiding incident, back in January. And it took another few months before she would tell me what lay behind that. Here, then, is the background.

The resentment among her fellow staff nurses had been

a reaction to what they saw as her over-zealousness and ambition. Ill feeling was not rife, by any means: there would be a bad day every so often, usually triggered by some attempt of Christine's to improve care on the ward, and then everything would die down and the atmosphere would return to normal. There was one member of staff, however, with whom Christine regularly clashed.

Alice had come to Hamilton several years before as a care assistant with a disturbing record: she had already been moved from another ward in St Wenceslas after staff and relatives had complained about her treatment of patients. It seems very odd that she should have been kept on at all, but apparently someone in the hospital management was sympathetic towards her and gave her a second chance.

This was not good news for the patients on Hamilton. Alice was often impatient with them, shouting at them for eating messily, telling confused patients they were stupid and sometimes even slapping them. At first many of the nurses took issue with her but, though she would stop what she was doing at the time, she would go on to repeat it on other occasions. She simply didn't seem to recognize what was wrong with her behaviour and most of the staff nurses gave up trying to make an impression.

Christine wouldn't let things pass when they happened in front of her and had a long string of confrontations with Alice. She reported most of them to the ward manager, who supported her attempts to improve Alice's care, telling Christine in private that she would like to get rid of Alice altogether, but was typically reluctant to make a decisive move, either with Alice or with management. Christine would not go over her head to hospital management; she felt that she had to let the ward manager take the initiative.

Alice's treatment of the patients was not, perhaps, physically cruel. Christine was anxious to explain that her slaps were mere taps, which would not cause pain. But emotionally and mentally cruel she certainly was. Christine had heard her round on a client who was asking for her brother and tell her not to be so stupid, her brother had been dead for years. And she habitually treated the clients as though they were encumbrances to be got into their clothes, washed, fed and put back to bed again. It wasn't done out of deliberate unkindness, thought Christine; it was just that Alice had no concept of the clients as people, with feelings and the right to respect.

It seemed odd to me, listening to Christine's account of this, that the Hamilton nursing staff as a whole let this go on. My clear impression from going on the ward was that the nurses treated the clients with respect and in some cases affection. Yet many staff nurses simply gave up remonstrating with Alice, and even Christine, who remonstrated all the time and took her complaints to the ward manager, did not want to go to management herself.

The explanation seems to lie in the fact that the nurses feel divorced from the hospital's management and forgotten by the NHS at large. They are not valued by the NHS – they are in elderly care, which is a poor area of the service, and many of them are enrolled nurses, considered only semi-qualified. Now, of course, enrolled nurses are being phased out (if you can call immediate abolition of their posts phasing); but even three years ago, when the trouble with Alice was at its worst, the staff nurses on Hamilton knew perfectly well that they were considered semi-skilled. Their loyalty to one another was therefore very strong. There was an instinct among many of them to absorb Alice's bad care and try to preserve their ward's reputation, rather than make a fuss. Christine was reluctant to take a step which might cause Alice's dismissal, especially as the other nurses would blame her.

One incident brought the matter to a head for Christine. While the clients were eating lunch one day, Alice told one of them, a lady just a few days off her hundredth birthday, that she was eating disgustingly and was anti-social. Christine was in the day room but too far away to intervene; meanwhile, as Alice went on expressing her distaste, the relatives of other clients were listening in disbelief. Another staff nurse, nearer by, told Alice to stop it; the lady would be one of Alice's special clients the next week so she should develop a better attitude towards her. Alice bounced up and down on her chair and declared repeatedly: 'I won't have her! I won't have her!'

The relatives began to talk angrily to each other. One said that Alice wasn't fit to look after anyone, but Alice didn't seem to hear; she got up and left the room to wash a plate. Christine followed her and reiterated what the relative had said; then she went to the ward manager and said that they had to act. The ward manager agreed, prepared to tell Alice to go – and then acceded to the pleas of the other nurses to give her another chance. What the ward manager did not realize was that Alice was currently negotiating with management to renew her contract. A couple of weeks later, without consultation between the hospital management and the ward, Alice was given an indefinite contract on Hamilton.

That had been three years ago; since then, Christine said, her continuous attentions, the intermittent ones of the other staff nurses and the organizing of study days for all ward staff to improve and update care had changed Alice's practice for the better. 'It's not 100 per cent,' said Christine, 'but it's probably about 75 per cent better.'

However, the friction between Alice and Christine had continued throughout this time and spread on occasions to the other nurses, most of whom took Alice's side. This had helped to fuel the ill feeling at which Christine had earlier hinted. It had culminated in January, with the incident over the shoes. Alice was one of the people who knew who had taken them.

After that affair and Christine's insistence on a formal warning from the ward manager, Alice had behaved more civilly towards her. And Christine's willingness to help the other nurses with their personal assessments had mended bridges generally. All the same, a week before her official leaving, Christine acknowledged that it had been these problems with her colleagues that had made early retirement a relatively easy decision.

As Christine would not be leaving St Wenceslas altogether, she told her colleagues she didn't want a party or any great fuss. Naturally enough they ignored this and she was given a joint party with another nurse who was leaving. The staff also clubbed together to buy her a present, a china horse nearly three feet high, which she had recently admired in a shop. (In the run up to the party, her son was puzzled by a phone call from one of the nurses, asking if his mother had bought the horse yet.) Christine was touched by the gesture and put the horse in her sitting room.

The next week she was back at St Wenceslas for two six-hour shifts, as an agency nurse. (Agency nurses are often hired for shorter shifts, to save money.) She was working on Reynold, the ward across the corridor from Hamilton, so she was able to go and say hello to her old clients.

On Reynold, so many nurses had just taken 'voluntary' redundancy or retirement, that the ward was abandoning named nursing. Christine knew a couple of the patients from the reminiscence group (which she no longer attended) and she knew most of the staff who remained on the ward. In her opinion the care was not as good as on Hamilton, but she was resolved not to try and change things, even though she thought that named nursing could have been continued with a bit of energetic organization.

The work was much the same as she had been doing before, but without the responsibility of being a team leader. One good thing had emerged from her registering with the agency: she was not after all employed as an A grade. Upon hearing of her experience and qualifications, the agency had insisted that she be hired as a D grade (i.e. just one grade below her true level, rather than four) and St Wenceslas agreed.

I must stress that Christine has never expressed anything other than polite pleasure at being thus partially reinstated. When I asked her if she felt aggrieved at the hospital's original stance, she just smiled and said that the management had been trying to save money. But surely this little episode shows why so many NHS staff are disillusioned and angry. When her hospital employers initially offered Christine the 'A' grade remuneration, were they trying to exploit her? Or were they simply fulfilling their duty under government rules to buy contractors' services as cheaply as possibly? And from Christine's standpoint, what exactly is the difference?

THROUGHOUT THE autumn, the adult branch students were busy. They were on new placements; they were all working towards the final exams in October and Corinne and Jane also did the resit of the summer nursing exam. This was held in early September and both were intensely nervous about it – with good reason, because if they failed a second time, they would probably be thrown off the course.

In the event, the paper was demanding but not terrifying. They both worked through the required number of questions and came out feeling that at least it was out of their hands. Corinne was slightly more sanguine than Jane, as she believed she had answered the questions more fully this time round. Jane was worried that she hadn't written enough. The results would not be out until early October, two weeks before the final exams.

By this stage, the students had covered most of the wards between them and were beginning to cross one another's tracks. The placements were now getting shorter again: this current one would run five weeks, stopping in October to allow them a week in college before the finals. Jane was now on ENT, Angela on Fussell general medical, Tim on Emerson, a high-dependency surgical ward. Emily was on Bartlett, the fantastically busy orthopaedic ward where Corinne had had her first ever ward experience, and Corinne was back at the Markham, on a private ward.

Corinne was disappointed to be going over old ground and complained to the college about it, but they told her that it was too late to change the placement. There was an advantage: the work was fairly undemanding, so she had plenty of energy left to revise. All the same, she would have preferred to be learning something new. True, she was on a mixed ward this time, but the patients were suffering from much the same conditions as those she had nursed in February, on the women's ward. What was more, as this was a private ward the patients were in individual rooms and a student would not normally go in unless the patient rang to request it. This cut down on the opportunity to talk to patients and to help out other nurses in the casual way common on NHS wards. Not that help was usually needed: staffing levels were good and skilled procedures like changing colostomy bags and stoma care tended to be done by registered nurses.

Corinne made the most of the chances she got to watch and learn, but she found the ward 'very quiet. The patients were very demanding though – you'd think we were servants rather than nurses. They'd complain about the littlest things. They'd say, "I'm paying £260 a night for this room and the service is terrible!" '

Nevertheless, Corinne got on well with the staff nurses and said that she was 'quite enjoying it'. This was characteristic of her: from the beginning she had been able to find something good in every placement. For instance, she had actually enjoyed being on Bartlett and now recalled it with enthusiasm. She liked to be busy, she said, and everyone had been rushed off their feet there. Being new to the wards, she hadn't been able to help as much as she wanted but 'it's the kind of ward I'd like if I was more experienced, qualified. They don't have enough staff there and the type of patients they have need a lot of care. At the time I had nothing to compare it to, but now, looking back, I think standards were definitely lower than they should be.'

Corinne's response to this was to think that here was a place where she could work and perhaps make a difference. Emily, who was currently on Bartlett, found the battle to maintain standards too gruelling. 'It's really disheartening to be allocated patients – maybe seven in the morning, in the afternoon it's usually nine – and to look at them all and know what they should have done, and not have time to do it. On so many wards it's been drummed into me that you should care for people as the care plan tells you to: make sure observations are done at a certain time, for instance. Yet sometimes you get to the end of the morning and all you've done is manage to get these people up, dressed, washed and comfortable. Observations which should have been done at 10 or 11 o'clock haven't been done, because there wasn't any time. It worries me, I do think it might be dangerous. There have been times when I've thought, this person might have a temperature but I wouldn't know about it unless they said to me, "I'm feeling hot." And ever since that man died of septic shock on Preston, I've always had it in the back of my mind that I might be missing things.'

Emily hated the feeling of going off duty knowing that there were things she hadn't done for the patients. The lack of psychological care bothered her too. 'Discharge planning tended not to be done properly. A lot of the clients are quite elderly and sometimes need a lot of explanations about their pills and things. They get quite confused. One lady who'd had a total knee replacement was being transferred to the

Wavetree (they needed her bed or something) and on the day she was due to leave she called to me just as I was about to go off and when I sat down she burst into tears and said she didn't know what was happening to her.'

Towards the end of the placement, a staff nurse took Emily aside and asked her to complain to the college about the low staffing on the ward. Emily was uncertain what to do: she didn't want to be labelled a troublemaker, nor did she want to criticize the sisters. As she approached the end of her time on Bartlett, she was trying to think up a diplomatic form of words for her placement evaluation. She was also feeling a huge sense of relief.

Even so, it hadn't been all bad. Or so she was able to acknowledge, with the worst of it safely behind her. 'It's given me an opportunity to put into practice some of what I've learnt about prioritizing care and actually see that I could keep my head above water when the manure was hitting the fan.'

This sense of consolidating what they had learnt and growing more confident was shared by all five students on the adult branch. Angela was surprising herself by enjoying her time on Fussell. As a general medical ward, it admitted patients with conditions from diabetes to eczema, alcoholism to strokes, so the nursing care was both varied and heavy. Staffing levels were (once again) poor, but despite the fact that she often felt she was on a treadmill of basic nursing care – lifting, bathing, clearing up after incontinent patients – Angela found herself warming to the ward.

'The staff are what make it. It's poorly staffed in terms of numbers but everyone is down to earth and they laugh all the time and make jokes out of things, even though the Alf's attitude is usually to be very serious. The sister has been there ten years – it's really rare to find that. She's very dedicated. And there are quite a few Scottish staff nurses. I really like their sense of humour.'

For the first time, Angela felt that she was truly part of a team. She also had a personal triumph with one of the patients: Flossie, who was in her sixties and diabetic and had come in for a leg amputation. Flossie was the kind of patient nurses either love or hate; she was physically tiny, raucous and rude. She hated being in hospital and demanded to be allowed to go home. But she had no concept of how to look after herself by eating a restricted diet and she was incontinent – in Angela's opinion, wilfully so. 'She'll go in the bed, then ring the nurse and tell her. It's the type of incontinence that's really hard to deal with because it's psychological rather than pathological. It's habitual – she's attention seeking.'

Perversely, Angela felt a great admiration for Flossie. She admired her fighting spirit and decided to try and harness it: she set herself the goal of making Flossie continent. 'I told her she wouldn't be allowed to go home until she achieved continence. I built up a really good rapport with her and it worked – she stopped going in the bed. I used to take her to the toilet and transfer her but she's now become more independent in washing herself and so forth. She's at the point where she can transfer from the wheelchair to the toilet without any assistance whatsoever.'

It was exhilarating to have made such an impact and to see Flossie finally discharged to go home. 'On Thursday 23rd, At Nine O'Clock In The Morning! You have to tell her that so many times a day; she's sure that we're all lying to her.'

It was the first time I had ever heard Angela talk about nursing with such warmth. It seemed that she was at last deriving some real satisfaction out of it. The sheer weight of work on Fussell cut through the hierarchy prevalent on some wards and made it possible for Angela to feel she belonged.

Moreover, time was starting to go quickly for her. As she approached the end of the placement, she felt that she was turning into the home straight. She was looking forward to going home once the course was finished in March, and as a consequence she was beginning to organize her impressions of her time at Alf's. Despite all the problems, she held the NHS in exasperated affection. 'It's definitely been worth it – working for the NHS has been one of the best experiences of my life. Because people really are treated so equally and in the States we don't have that sense of equal access to health care. And also the total hilarity of the NHS: all those confused patients wandering around, having a ball in these twenty-six-bed wards. All these men with amputations having political arguments and telling each other to shut up! You wouldn't find it anywhere else.'

She was already feeling nostalgic for it, anticipating a very different way of working in America. But the premonitory pang was nothing compared to the prospect of being back with Mark, both of them earning and leading a regular, adult independent life. 'It'll be the first time since we've been together,' she said with relish.

The autumn placement also made Jane feel more settled with nursing as a career. She liked the staff on the ENT ward, describing them as 'the nicest bunch I've ever worked with. They seem more mature than some of the others.' The ward had more outliers (overflow patients from other wards) than ever in September, so she was seeing patients with conditions like strokes and colostomies as well as the usual ENT conditions. She struck up a good relationship with one man who'd had a stroke; they talked and joked in a deadpan way, sharing the same sense of humour.

But like Angela, Jane intended to leave the NHS; she felt more strongly than ever that she couldn't and wouldn't accept the NHS culture. 'It's not just the money. It's the attitudes of the nurses and staff ... which is probably to do with there not being any money.' Even the nice staff on the ENT ward were, in her opinion, 'pissy' about such things as time-keeping. She didn't see what they could expect when they put people on eight-day stretches of duty: 'As far as I'm concerned, if you tire people out like that, you can't expect them not to oversleep.' She thought she would apply to the Navy when she registered. 'I want a job with security, where I won't have to worry about money.'

Tim, meanwhile, had every intention of applying to work in the NHS and was busy steadily extending his ward experience to that end. His confidence was not so much growing as establishing itself in different settings. His first two weeks on Emerson nearly swept him off his feet. Full of high-dependency patients just out of major surgery for things like embolisms and amputations, the ward was very busy, understaffed and run in an atmosphere of frantic tail-chasing. 'They were running about trying to do half a dozen jobs at once and getting nowhere. It was "Do this," then "Leave it and do that." At first I did, but then after two weeks I calmed down and decided to complete each job properly before going on to the next.'

Emerson was run in a very old-fashioned way: the principal aim of the nurses seemed to be to spare the next shift work, so things were often done in a peculiar order. 'For instance the morning staff might try to get all the dressings done, so at 1 o'clock in the afternoon you'd have a patient lying in an unmade bed, not washed, but with his dressings done. The care itself was good, but it was sometimes the wrong way round and it didn't work for the staff or the patients.'

Another manifestation of the old-fashioned approach was that whenever doctors came on the ward 'they're treated like gods. Because we have general and vascular surgery patients, there are several consultancy teams and five or six doctors' rounds in a week. Everything stops for them. I don't see the point of it. The doctor is as much a part of the team in patient care as we are; they shouldn't expect it.'

On every ward he worked on, Tim always noticed the way the doctors behaved. This is probably because hospital doctors are still a predominantly male bunch; the fact that they enjoy a higher status in hospitals than (predominantly female) nurses is simply a reflection of the higher status men have in society at large. Women may object to this but they are scarcely surprised by it. To Tim, however, it was very noticeable. He lacked the social conditioning which makes women accustomed to being deferential to men simply because the men expect it. When doctors of either gender assumed that the nurses were there to look up to them, he objected.

Tim observed the spiralling efforts of the nurses on Emerson with interest. He decided that the sister was responsible for much of the sense of pressure and that other staff were picking it up. He thought that good organization could have lifted the load from the ward and his impression was confirmed when two new E grade staff nurses started work towards the end of the placement. They both had experience on similar wards and went about their work calmly, making a difference straight away.

Organization (or the lack of it) apart, Tim enjoyed working with surgical patients because for many of them there was a clear progression from illness to recovery. He didn't rule out the idea of applying to work on Emerson when he registered: 'I'd look on it as a challenge. I wouldn't go in there all guns blazing but I would have my own team of patients and be responsible for them, so I could do the things I wanted to do for them and gradually say to other people, "I've done this. It seems to be working; why don't you try it?" '

At the beginning of October, Jane and Corinne heard that they had passed the resits. Barely ten days later, the autumn placements ended and all of the original Project 2000 intake who had made it this far (seventy-six out of seventy-eight) crammed into a last week's lectures and classes in the college before sitting the final exams.

*

DURING THE RUN UP to these exams, Rachel was doing her second (and last) rostered service placement on Walsh, the children's oncology ward. She had arrived there at the very end of August, with four colleagues. The ten child branch students, who were divided into two groups for placement purposes, had done a straight swap of wards: she and the other four who had spent summer on Howard went downstairs to Walsh; the five from Walsh switched to Howard. Rachel's group was nervous about the move: from the other students' accounts, the work on Walsh was heavier and more specialized than anything they were used to. And the Walsh group spoke about the ward with an almost possessive enthusiasm, which Rachel and her friends wondered if they could match.

None of the students had been down to Walsh on the weekend shifts; they had been told that the work was too specialized for them to be able to pick up on one or two visits. So when they began their placement, they had no illusions and plenty of apprehensions.

Rachel's first impression was of a large ward, somewhat dark and divided into bays like Howard. Although the physical layout was similar, everything was kept in a different place and the nurses seemed to be moving continuously between patients, parents and various pieces of equipment. Obviously very busy, the staff tried to take the new students on board quickly, co-opting them into the round of observations and basic care. Rachel spent the first days desperately trying to orientate herself. 'It's difficult. The staff are used to the other lot, who know their way around and we really don't know anything. Everything's different here – the paper work, the care plans. And the cancers themselves – they're just all so complicated.'

Walsh has twenty-three beds, only eighteen of which were in use. Rachel didn't know why, but assumed that the ward lacked the money to staff the others: the nurses were spread pretty thin as it was. Of the eighteen beds available, ten were almost always full and sometimes all eighteen were taken. Their occupancy was in a continuous state of change as children came on to the ward for chemotherapy or for treatment of infections and went home again, sometimes staying only one night.

The patients were aged from babyhood up to eighteen. Most of them knew the ward well as they had been coming here for months or even years. Walsh treats many different kinds of cancer. It is England's specialist centre for retinoblastoma, an eye tumour, and most of the babies Rachel saw were suffering from this. A high proportion of the patients had acute lymphoblastic leukaemia (ALL), which is a common form of cancer in children; others had bone cancer and cancer of the nervous system. There were also some children with cancers usually associated with adults: a three-year-old girl with acute myeloid leukaemia and a boy of seventeen with cancer of the testicles.

During the first week, Rachel was extremely busy with basic nursing tasks; this meant doing observations, getting children dressed or undressed, washed and fed and keeping the ward clean and tidy. Meanwhile, through reading care plans when she had the time and asking questions of the staff when she thought they had the time, she built up a picture of how Walsh operated.

When a child is first diagnosed with cancer at Alf's, he or she is usually admitted at once and stays two or three weeks on Walsh, having initial treatment to try to bring the disease under control. Depending on the type of cancer, this might be chemotherapy, surgery or radiotherapy. Once this is finished, the child usually returns home to rest and build up strength before coming back in for further treatment, which aims to get the cancer into remission.

'Further treatment' can mean radiotherapy and/or chemotherapy; most of the children Rachel saw on the ward were being treated with chemotherapy.

Chemotherapy is given intravenously, via IV 'machines': electronically operated drip apparatuses. Almost all the children have Hickman lines. Rachel had vaguely imagined bays full of silent, wasted children lying strapped to their machines, but the reality was different: many of the children were quite well and full of energy, despite the disease, and half of those having chemotherapy on any one day were likely to be up and about, wheeling their machines with them.

Each child's chemotherapy is specific to the nature and stage of the disease, so children receive different drugs in varying combinations and strengths. Some might come in for one day; others will stay a week. Chemotherapy has a dehydrating effect, so as part of the treatment children are rehydrated with intravenous fluid drips; monitoring their fluid intake is an important part of the nursing care.

Not all children who come in do so to receive chemotherapy itself; some are admitted with infections which have developed after chemotherapy. Because chemotherapy destroys fast-growing cells in the body, it lowers children's resistance to infection. Therefore, if children develop high temperatures or other signs of infection when they are at home, their parents bring them back in for observation and treatment, usually with antibiotics.

As a student, Rachel was not supposed to touch the IV machines. But her work involved continuous and important observations, to check that they were working properly, as well as a heavy routine of general nursing care.

'If there are children in having chemotherapy, you have a lot of set observations and tasks you have to do throughout the day. You get in, say, on an early and have handover. You get allocated to work with somebody, or a few people, perhaps a bay. Then what I usually do is go round my patients and write down what each of them individually needs. Because in handover you write down the needs of everyone, which is a lot to remember, and if I didn't sort out my own patients specially I'd spend all day going and looking at their charts, because I'd have forgotten what I needed to do for them. And when I'm taking notes about them, I say "hi".

'They usually need medicines at about 9 o'clock so I toddle off and prepare their drugs on a tray and get a staff nurse to come and check them.

'Depending on whether their parents are there the next thing is to get them up and generally tidy up the ward. If they've got fluid going into them intravenously, as part of the chemo, you have to read the machines every hour. And because they've got so much fluid going in, they're all on fluid balance charts, so you have to weigh every child and measure everything that's coming out to make sure that they're not retaining fluid and they're not dehydrated. The parents are really well trained and know how to label all the bottles of urine and leave them in the sluice and you have to go in and measure all the urines, and note them down and get rid of them – you do that when you haven't got anything else to do.

'You check what they're eating and drinking. They're quite lively. Hardly any of them are sick, because they're given good anti-sickness drugs. They're generally quite well.

'You check the machines every hour, and then you have your observations at 11 o'clock, which are temperature, blood pressure, pulse and resps (respiratory rate).

'And you have to do mouth assessments on them. Because the chemo kills off rapidly growing cells, hence the hair falling out, so it is with the mucous membranes. So you check their mouths. It's really important for them: they're all on mouth care and have mouth washes and a liquid they have to swallow to prevent the mouth from breaking down. Otherwise they get mouth ulcers and cracked lips; it's really bad – on their tongues, bleeding gums. You have to score the appearance of their mouth on a chart: if it's pink and normal inside and their saliva's watery, it's fine. You have to encourage them to do their mouth care because if they get sore mouths, they don't eat and they weaken.

'And apart from all these tasks that you have to do, the phone's always ringing with queries, and another parent will ask you to do so-and-so, and in between times you're trying to empty the linen sacks, or put the washing on, or put it into the drier. There's always something. It is a very heavy day's work.'

For the first few weeks, Rachel badly missed the mentor system which had operated on Howard; here there was simply no time for it. And on several occasions she and her fellow students found themselves uncertain as to what they were and were not allowed to do.

'There were days when there was only one qualified nurse on the ward and if, for instance, a machine was alarming to say that the fluid bag was running out, we would top it up. We knew how to do it, but strictly speaking we thought we shouldn't be doing it. It was very confusing actually. We asked in college about it and the college didn't really know either.'

She also had the impression that the staff nurses would have been happy for her to go ahead and do things that were definitely supposed to be out of a student's province, such as giving out drugs. As it was, though, she limited herself to 'drawing up' the antibiotics (setting them out on the tray) and then asking a qualified nurse to come and check them.

Rachel and the other students were sympathetic to the staff nurses, who were under constant strain because their numbers were too low, but they decided that they would take no risks.

There were good days and bad days. As Rachel got to know the staff, the children and their families, she began to enjoy the work and feel quite deeply attached to the ward. She saw children she had met at the start of the placement come back in again and developed particular friendships with some of them.

One was Mandy, the three-year-old with acute myeloid leukaemia, rarely found in children. She was having a particularly strong form of chemotherapy and suffering from the associated side effects: her hair fell out, she developed serious infections and at one stage she was so ill that she went into heart failure. She survived and responded to treatment, but Rachel said that everything about Mandy 'pulls at my heartstrings. She's so used to hospital – you go to do her blood pressure and she just gives me her arm. And she's so quiet. She doesn't talk much for her age anyway, but when she's very sick she completely clams up and stops communicating.'

Mandy was in and out of Walsh very often, for chemotherapy and to have the associated illnesses treated. Rachel got to know her family well and was astonished by how well they coped. 'But then they all do. It's amazing how they get through something so mind-blowing.'

The other patient Rachel was drawn to was Rick, the seventeen-year-old. He had developed cancer of the testicles at fourteen after being kicked in the groin during a rugby match. The cancer had gone into remission and he had been clear of it for a time, but now it had reappeared and the prognosis wasn't good. Rachel talked to Rick, not about his illness which he didn't really discuss, but about his interests and his plans.

'He's got nine, ten O levels [GCSEs]; he did them while he was in hospital and passed them. He wants to do A levels, he wants to go to university. He's realized what his potential is and he also understands the full extent of his illness and the fact that he probably isn't going to make it. I don't know if he's officially been told that, but I think he knows it. And the whole family is so nice and so close and that makes it even harder. His sister's just gone to university. They all talk to me – oh, it just makes me cry. And sometimes it makes me really angry.'

By the end of September the students felt much more

sympathetic towards the staff nurses on Walsh, as they could see how much stress their work laid on them. The students felt it too, especially now as the final exam approached and they had to try and fit revision in with their shifts.

The need to work for the exam was underlined rather cruelly when one of Rachel's flatmates, who had failed the summer exam, learned that she had failed the resit too. It was a complete shock to her, followed by an even greater one when the college was as good as its word and told her she was off the course. She put in an appeal, which would take some time to go through, but meanwhile her future looked pretty grim. She was terribly upset and for several weeks she stayed in the flat crying. Rachel and the others took it in turns to comfort her and tried to do their revision as discreetly as possible.

'It's so difficult; since we've moved in we've become really close, the four of us. I felt I couldn't just shut myself in my room and work when she was sitting in the living room sobbing her heart out. And we used to grumble to each other about the pressure of revision in secret, but we all knew that she'd love to be coping with it.'

Then one of the other girls heard that her grandmother had died; all in all, the month running up to the exam was not a good one. In the end it was almost a relief to sit the paper, especially when it turned out to be quite straight-forward. Like the nurses on the adult branch, they felt they had acquitted themselves reasonably well but there was a distinct lack of jubilation in the air, perhaps because they would have to wait till Christmas for the results.

After the exam, Rachel had a last couple of weeks on Walsh. To her slight surprise, she blossomed during them: with the worry about revision lifted, she was able to concentrate on the work and she realized that she had learnt a lot.

'I know now that I *can* look after seven patients on a shift, because I've done it. I've gained a hell of a lot of experience and clinical skill. And now I think we all appreciate what a lot of stress the staff are under, so we don't wait to be asked, we say, "Will you show me what to do?" and try to help them. And they've really accepted us. When I go on the ward now I love seeing them all and having a laugh and a joke.'

Just before Rachel left, she heard good news about Mandy. She had recovered well enough to go home and hadn't been in at all for the last few weeks; now her parents had brought her in for a lumbar puncture, to assess the state of the cancer cells, and none had shown up: she was in remission.

This did not mean she was cured of course; remissions can be of varying lengths. But for the time being, she was free of the disease, when Rachel had half expected that she might have to cope with seeing her die.

Chemotherapy does not necessarily cease when a patient is in remission, and on Rachel's last shift, she found Mandy back on the ward for another session. But it was a much livelier, healthier Mandy: her hair had grown back and she was chatting freely. It was a weekend shift, the first weekend in November, and fireworks were being set off across the city. In the early evening, Rachel sat by the window with Mandy, talking and watching them explode. Later that night she sat and played cards with Rick.

It was a rare shift on Walsh, one where she had the time to talk and listen as much as the children (and adolescents) needed. She thought that despite everything she would like to come back.

Winter

NICOLA'S FEELINGS about the Grange had always been ambivalent. She had enjoyed her placement there almost one year ago and, in all her subsequent time in the hospitals, clinics and housing estates of Wavetree, she had thought of it as a model, well-resourced hospital, the kind of place to which everyone should have access. Not everything she had come across there last year had been perfect (the doctors' readiness to use ECT, for instance, had troubled her) but there was no denying that the environment was superb, the nursing care good, and the resources such that patients actually received the attention and support they needed.

Her reservations sprang from the fact that the Grange was private. It took NHS patients, usually on referral from GPs, but only a few, generally patients whose condition would respond to short-term treatment. It was clear to Nicola, from what she had seen on her NHS placements, that private concerns like the Grange would never meet the needs of the large numbers of long-term mentally ill people. No matter how many Granges came into being, and how diligently health authorities bought their services, they would not make much of an impression on the real problem. Like most successful enterprises, they were concerned to concentrate on the profitable end of the market: treating the treatable patients, especially those with private health insurance.

All the same, from the point of view of her training, the Grange offered the chance to take part in mental health nursing at its best. Nicola had therefore put her reservations to one side and opted to do her elective placement there.

She began in November, feeling in better spirits than when she had left the Link. Her father was getting stronger and her worry for him had eased. She had managed to take the final exams along with the rest of her set and, having done so, was glad that she had got them out of the way. She had spent some of her two weeks' holiday at home and some in London with David. She was refreshed and looking forward to the next two months.

The Grange was a small hospital which was well furnished and tended, rather like an upper-range country hotel. The ground floor had been turned into a thirty-bed general ward, with individual bedrooms, a few bays, two day rooms, a dining room and consulting rooms. Patients were admitted on to this ward with illnesses that included depression, obsessive compulsive disorder and psychosis. The Grange also had two specialist units on the upper floor: an Eating Disorders Unit and an Alcohol Treatment Unit. These both took a small number of in-patients and a larger number of day patients.

'There's a very extensive therapy programme. People on the general ward either go into a cognitive-behavioural therapy programme, where they go to groups every day, or they go to a programme organized by the occupational therapist. Outside therapists often come in to give these – there's creative writing, psychodrama, art therapy; the programmes are quite full. People at the Eating Disorders Unit and the Alcohol Treatment Unit have their own programmes, attending groups and sometimes having one-to-one therapy.

'The nurses on the wards, whether it's the general ward or one of the units, aren't involved in the groups. They just do day-to-day care which makes their role quite limited. But I want to spend some time on a ward because I need to get my drugs up to scratch. I'm here with another girl from my set, Melanie, and we asked if we could each divide our time between the general ward and one of the specialities.'

Melanie was allocated a place on the general ward and, as

there were students already attached to occupational and cognitive-behavioural therapy, Nicola was offered the chance to go to the Eating Disorders Unit. She accepted, but when she turned up to start work, she found that the patients were reluctant to let her in.

'It was awful. Everyone on the unit gets involved in small groups which are a prelude to the psychotherapy that some of them will be going on to. The groups are for identifying feelings, talking about them, why you're ill, family relationships – anything and everything really. They tend to be close, intimate groups. I was supposed to be going into one of these. But they didn't want me. They were so defensive, they thought an outsider wouldn't understand, would judge them, wouldn't keep their confidence. The nurse-therapist had been asking them for the two weeks before I started if I could join and they said no. Then for the first week that I was here they still said no.'

Nicola spent a miserable first week, trying to learn about the work of the unit from the staff and by reading up the literature. In her second week, the members of the group reluctantly agreed to allow her in.

'They were very, very suspicious of me. I gave a little introduction and said that I'd had a friend who'd been hospitalized for anorexia nervosa (which was true), that eating disorders were quite common among nurses, so I had an idea what it was all about, and that it would be very useful for me for my training.'

The ice didn't exactly melt, but the five members of the group accepted her presence, albeit warily. The group was meeting three times a week. Nicola attended each meeting, taking things slowly and carefully, listening hard.

Because the issues of trust and confidentiality were so important for these patients, Nicola did not want to describe the exact make-up of the group, or give exact times for when things happened. She ended up staying eight weeks on the

Eating Disorders Unit and came to know a number of different patients.

'The two main disorders people have are anorexia and bulimia. With anorexia, you restrict or completely stop eating and have a distorted body image. You starve yourself, or sometimes you eat and then purge yourself. With bulimia you have bingeing, then you purge yourself through laxatives, vomiting or fasting. Some anorexics binge but in smaller quantities, because the body can't accept the amount of food. Anorexics lose weight, sometimes to a dangerous extent; bulimics tend to be normal weight or slightly overweight.

'We have room for twelve in-patients and most of them are anorexics and young – fourteen to twenty-one. They are all here "voluntarily" at the moment, though I would imagine there's been a fair bit of coercion from some of the families. Some of them are very ill. One girl came in at 4½ stone. She couldn't walk.'

All the patients were female, except for one young man who was bulimic. Eating disorders commonly affect women more than men: the reasons for this are thought to be connected to women's and girls' lack of influence in society. On the receiving end of numerous pressures about how to look and behave, some women and girls try to exert control in the only way they feel is open to them: by regulating what goes into their bodies.

From what was said in the groups, it became overwhelmingly clear to Nicola that these pressures were to be found in one form in society at large; in others within the patients' own families. 'They talk a lot about their families and we call family meetings to discuss the problems and how the parents relate to the children. I can't think of one of our patients' families which is really healthy. They tend to be very over-involved, intrusive. There doesn't tend to be much of a boundary between people: you know, everyone's enmeshed. Anorexia's very much about control over oneself.

'There's often a history of sexual abuse and then the anorexia can be a form of denial of sexuality. And there's often been a kind of emotional abuse: the child is used as a confidante much sooner than they should be.'

This was the case with one girl whom Nicola took on as a special patient: 'I'll call her Joanne. She's fourteen, though at first she came across as a thirty-year-old, she was so mature and controlled. She's got a very strange father who's got psychiatric problems: for a long time he'd been abusive and violent and moody. And her mother (who's actually a very senior nurse) was using Joanne to offload all her problems and discuss the father endlessly – had been doing it for years. Last year the father had a heart attack and became quite pathetic as well as difficult and it was all too much for Joanne, That was when she developed anorexia.

'She was lucky in that her condition was caught quite early. She wasn't dangerously low weight when she came in and she still knew what normal eating was. At her first assessment, she immediately started talking about her father. We heard a lot about him for the first few weeks, but since then the anger about her mother is coming out. The mother didn't protect her, the mother used her, why had she been deprived of a happy childhood? She's really, really angry and she's starting to act more like a teenager – she slams doors and stamps her foot. It's good. She's adamant now that she won't go back home, so we're looking into boarding schools for her.'

Joanne's anorexia was still at a relatively early stage and she was bringing herself back to normal eating patterns quite quickly. She was also addressing the underlying problems directly. Some of the other people at the unit were in a much worse state, such as Heidi, the girl who had come in weighing $4\frac{1}{2}$ stone.

'At first she was quite mad. She was seeing things crawling up the walls and over the floor. She imagined people wanted to harm her physically. For the first two weeks, while she was being nursed on a liquid diet, she thought the anorexia had come out of the blue. She'd say, "We're a very close family, there's nothing wrong. This thing's just come over me." '

Once she began gaining weight, Heidi's hallucinations went and her fears lessened. She also began to hint at "a big secret in the family that I can't talk about". From her veiled allusions, the staff were beginning to suspect that she had been sexually abused by her elder brother. They would never prompt a disclosure like that, for fear of "leading" the patient, or of forcing her to confront the problem too early, so they were waiting for her to tell more in her own time. Meanwhile, Heidi was having difficulty accepting the prospect of normal eating. 'She's thinking that if she gets better, the family won't love her any more. She's twenty-one but she's the youngest child and still very attached to home; she can't bear the thought of separating.'

Patients such as Heidi often benefit from cognitive-behavioural therapy, which helps them look at the emotional reasons for why they aren't eating and disentangle the behaviour from all the things they associate with it. 'For instance, anorexics are often afraid to eat in front of their family, in case the family decides that everything's all right now. They really resent the idea of that. So they have to identify all the beliefs that are going with that, such as "They'll think I'm better. They won't notice me any more. I won't be special any more." Then they set themselves tasks, such as to have one meal with the family.'

Nicola found the EDU's work more interesting than she had expected, especially since she had been able to concentrate on the therapeutic side. There was a general nursing aspect to the unit: the nurses who worked on the unit's ward gave basic nursing care and supervised the patients' diet. 'They are on a strict regime, they have to be. Those who come in dangerously underweight go on liquid diets; others are on a regimented schedule of eating and the nurses have to take them to the dining room, supervise their meals and give them physical care. The ward nurses don't get involved in the groups at all.'

The nurses working in the groups were all psychiatric nurses and were distinguished from their counterparts on the ward by being called 'counsellors'. The title wasn't strictly accurate, but it was useful for the patients and gave a fair indication of the therapy-driven nature of the work. Nicola enjoyed it and her inclination towards this kind of work strengthened: when the time came to switch from the EDU to the general ward, she was really sorry to go and was delighted when the people in the group told her they would be sorry to lose her. On many of her placements, the staff had been complimentary about her but to hear this from the patients, who had been so defensive at the start, meant a great deal. 'The staff can look at what you do from the outside, but the patients are the only ones who know how it feels.'

Even so, she was taken aback when, as she was preparing to leave for the Christmas break, the unit offered her a job. The counsellor who ran cognitive-behavioural therapy was going on maternity leave soon; Nicola was invited to fill the vacancy when she registered.

She had four days to think about it. She discussed it with David; she rang her parents and talked it over with them. She had not expected to take her first job outside the NHS and had a struggle to justify it to herself. But she could not think of any very good reason for refusing so, after a quiet Christmas at home with her parents, she rang the Grange and accepted.

IN OCTOBER, Catherine and Bob finally escaped together for their holiday. They went to Portugal on a last-minute booking and had a long-overdue lazy time. Catherine recovered from the exigencies of her early months at the Link; Bob from the scramble and hustle of applying for jobs in the community. They set off on the return journey feeling rested; twenty-four hours later, after a mix up over plane tickets had finally been sorted out, they arrived back in London somewhat less rested. Half an hour after Catherine had got back inside her house, the telephone rang and she heard that one of her close friends had committed suicide.

'I knew she was depressed,' Catherine said some time afterwards, 'but obviously, I didn't realize she was that low. She did it while we were away, on Bob's birthday actually. So while we were celebrating, she was doing that. It's not a date I'm ever likely to forget now.'

Inevitably, all the things that go with such an event began to manifest themselves: not just the grief but the bewilderment, the self-reproach, the picking over with hindsight. Catherine went to the funeral and met the other friends. They arranged to meet again before Christmas, which was something they did most years, but this year it would be a kind of memorial.

Going back to work was quite a relief. At least the Link was a place where personal bereavements could be acknowledged, and Catherine was now sufficiently settled to find comfort in her work, which she felt she was doing well.

She was still doing the same groups and had developed the relaxation theory group in particular so that it had become her baby. It was now more sophisticated, she felt, with clients not only learning the background to relaxation but investigating the different techniques and discovering which suited them best. It was proving popular and she'd had some encouraging feedback.

She was taking on more clients: ten rather than six. Among these and the clients attending her groups were several who had been at the Link in the summer and were now back for another cycle. Victor was there, making great strides: he was still nervous and anxious but he no longer heard his mother's voice and was able to see that what she had told him about women was not necessarily true.

'Bless his heart! He's still got a lot of problems but he's streets ahead of where he was. In the men's group, he can now say, "My mother brought me up in a way that has made it very difficult for me to have relationships with women." He's reaching out to people and making friendships. He's such a kind, generous man that you can't help but like him. People are very fond of him and I think that's been great for him.'

Elizabeth, the woman whose son had died, was still there too; she was a tough customer with layers of defence built up over the course of a hard life but she was opening up gradually. On this second cycle she was talking more and, largely thanks to her, the women's group had shed the worst of its long silences. She told Catherine that she felt cared for at the Link. As the second cycle went on, she began to act almost like an elder in the groups, helping others to talk and even coming to Catherine's rescue. 'If things aren't going right, she'll get the group going. She'll get me out of trouble sometimes.'

Elizabeth had always been one of Catherine's special clients and Catherine had become fond of her; this was a measure of how her own confidence had grown because, she admitted sheepishly, at first she had been quite frightened of her. 'She's a very prickly woman. She's very tough and physically big, she's quite bolshy. At the beginning I thought, "Oh-h-h!" But now I just like her. When her son died, as she says, her reason for living went. But she's here, and I admire her courage and her spirit to carry on.'

Catherine's second full cycle of groups ended in mid-November. Elizabeth was going to come back for a third time, not because she was in dire need of the groups, but because the Link was succeeding where everything else had failed and both she and the staff were loath to sever contact. Victor, on the other hand, was very keen to be discharged.

'He wants to end with a big bang and go out into the world. But John feels very strongly that it would be too drastic for him, so he's been persuaded to keep coming here on a very reduced programme: just one day a week.'

Now that she had the chance to take stock, Catherine realized that although she felt happy at the Link and confident about her work, she was still habitually exhausted. She went to her GP and asked to have some tests done and the results showed that the post-viral condition which she'd had earlier in the year was still there. 'At least it's something physical. It's a combination really: there's this underlying post-viral thing and the fact that I was pushing myself so hard when I first came to the Link. The trouble is that there's no clear treatment for it.' Various holistic and herbal remedies were being suggested, along with instructions to get plenty of rest.

That, however, seemed unlikely. Her new caseload was a heavy one. It included Simon, an extremely shy, almost socially phobic young man who had already been to the Link two years before. Back then he had become entangled with a female client who was by all accounts very clever and articulate, the very things Simon felt he was not. This woman was married and Simon had proceeded to have a long, impassioned and finally inconclusive affair with her. Eventually she had told him she would not leave her husband but as far as Catherine could gather, the relationship continued. Simon's confidence had taken a further battering from this and so he had presented himself to the Link again.

Ilana, the depressed woman whose father had died, and who had enrolled at the Link in July, had also reappeared. She had not come to many groups on her original cycle, but this time she made a big effort to attend. It cost her – even the way she sat expressed pain – but Catherine was encouraged that she was able to take part.

Then there was Trisha, who lived inside her head, forever analysing the way she and the world interacted. Trisha had been an alcoholic and seemed reluctant to become too closely involved in the groups. She did not turn up at all in the third week of the cycle. Catherine established through repeated phone calls that she had been drinking again.

Catherine also had one very unusual case: Penny, in her mid-twenties, was actually an in-patient on a St Wenceslas ward. She had been ill for two years and had received attention from an assortment of agencies. None had been able to do her much good and after each intervention she was left, in Catherine's words, 'walking round the table at home, chanting to try and keep her brain together'. She had now had a CAT scan, and the initial signs were that she was suffering from some kind of degenerative disease which affected the brain. Penny didn't know the diagnosis; at the moment her energies were concentrated on resisting going home. 'She lives with her mother who's very good at drawing people in to try and help. Penny's a bit better now than she was and she thinks she'll deteriorate again if she goes home.' No one knew at the moment exactly what Penny's diagnosis was and how much her improvement owed to drugs and physical care. It was extremely unusual for the Link to accept an in-patient, but Penny had had such a terrible time for the last two years that they were making an exception for her. Catherine anticipated a lot of work.

After three weeks of the cycle, there was a break. It was the week before Christmas and the Link gave its staff and clients a week off from formal groups. Instead the staff held morning meetings to plan their objectives for the next year and to discuss the ways in which the Link might develop as part of Wavetree's community care. In the afternoons the clients came in for board games, charades and general run-up-to-Christmas socializing.

It was a structured change of tempo, typical of the way the Link operated, the kind of thing Catherine would have been inclined to criticize six months before, or at least look at askance. Now she vigorously endorsed it. 'The thing is, people don't really know what we do here. I didn't before I came. I had all sorts of fantasies about the place. I thought it was a bit indulgent, dealing with the worried well. What surprised me was how unwell all the people were who came here. I suppose compared to some acute patients on the ward they are well but they are also very demanding, with high expectations.

'I do come across disparaging attitudes towards the Link among other mental health nurses and I think, "Well crikey, come and work here for a bit then!" I think half the nursing population would sink without trace if they tried it.'

Catherine was sure that she was not going to sink. On the contrary, she felt that she had a future here. 'I still find the structure oppressive to a certain degree, but I've found space within it to be me. I'm not trying to fit in with everyone else any longer, not always trying to be professional and serious . . .' The original six months she had promised herself to stay were almost over and she was now planning to stay at least another six, probably longer. She said she had learnt 'an incredible amount' since she had been at the Link and judged that she was developing good skills for moving out into other community jobs in the future.

She did not yet feel as fond of the Link staff as she did of her friends on Wilcox. In the week before Christmas she went to the Wilcox staff party and was reminded of how much she missed them all. But she seemed, and said that she felt, much more settled and at peace with herself than at this time last year.

Against the odds it had turned into a good year professionally. There had been a dark side, however: the death of her friend (the Christmas reunion was now just a few days away) and her own insidious physical illness. She had little doubt that the frantic work and stress of the summer had brought the post-viral syndrome back on and she was uneasy about it, because she couldn't see how to make herself well. She described it as a 'spectre'.

Though tired, she was optimistic about the coming year. She had two main hopes concerning it: that Bob would get a job in the community too and that her health would improve, so that when they eventually had free time to spend together, she would be fit enough to enjoy it.

BACK IN NOVEMBER with the final exams behind them, and refreshed to a greater or lesser degree by their two weeks' break, the adult branch students had begun the last part of their course. Between November and March they would each go on three more placements: they would be shorter, lasting between four and six weeks, and the students would once more be supernumerary. For most students, the three would include a stint in A & E, a community placement and their elective.

Electives, where students choose their own placement, have long been one of the more enjoyable parts of training, for nurses and doctors alike. Medical students very often go abroad for them and everyone on the course seemed to know nurses who had in the past done the same. This year, however, Alf's adult branch students had been invited to choose from a fairly small selection of options. Each set was offered a slightly different range: the students in this book could choose theatres, day surgery, AIDS, renal or ITU.

Project 2000 was partly responsible for the narrowness of the choice: students had to do their placements on wards which had been vetted as suitable for the course and could meet the needs of the curriculum. Given the shortage of other hospitals running Project 2000, this effectively meant that students had to work in Alf's itself, or one of its sister hospitals. Add to that the logistical problem of trying to co-ordinate the diverse choices of sixty third-year nursing students, and it becomes obvious why Alf's simplified matters by limiting choice.

Some on the adult branch felt they had had a raw deal. Compared to their counterparts on the mental health branch, they certainly had: while Nicola and her colleagues had to stay within the Wavetree Health Authority, they were still able to design placements to suit their own interests. On the other hand, Rachel and her colleagues on the child branch had no elective at all.

The list of elective options for the adult branch had gone up in September, to a mixed reception. Our five students reacted in varying, characteristic ways: Jane was angry and aggrieved, especially when she arrived at the list late to find that the only places left unselected were in theatres: 'a nightmare job. You're stuck in there, underground, all the time'. Angela was scathing and distinctly unexcited by any of the options; she put her name down for theatres because she was slightly frightened of working with unconscious people and thought this would be a good time to get over it. Emily remarked mildly that the list wasn't very extensive and put her name down for the AIDS unit; Tim was pleased to see that the renal unit was an option and promptly signed for it. Corinne just got on with choosing from what was there: she decided theatres would be interesting. 'It's definitely not what I want to do in the future, but I want to see what it's like.'

CORINNE STAYED in London for the two-week break. In the summer she had begun going out with a new man, Harry, and she spent most of her time off with him. She more or less moved out of the nurses' home and did not miss it at all.

The last stretch of the course began for her with the elective. She and her fellow students were assigned to theatres at the Wavetree and she went down on the first day feeling curious in a pleasantly unpressured sort of way.

There are four different theatre rooms at the Wavetree, all underground. (Theatres are usually underground; operations are done under bright, artificial light so there is no need for windows.) Each room has its own speciality: Theatre One is orthopaedics, Theatre Two obstetrics, Theatre Three general medical, including dental surgery, Theatre Four neurology.

At first, the students were told, they would be allowed only to watch operations. After a few weeks, they would be able to work as scrub nurses. Corinne was disappointed: she preferred doing to watching and had been looking forward to a busy, useful placement. But when the operations began, there was so much to observe and try and absorb, that she began to be grateful for the long introduction.

'There are usually about five nurses and support staff in the theatre, a scrub nurse, who assists the surgeon, and a runaround nurse. There's a porter who makes sure all the equipment is working. Sometimes the sister is there. And there might be some students.

'As a scrub nurse you have to make sure you're sterile, because you're working in a sterile environment. First you go into the scrub room to wash your hands: there's a procedure for this – it should take five minutes just scrubbing away. Then once your hands are washed you have to put gloves on and then your green gown. Once that's done you're not allowed to touch anyone else because you are supposed to be sterile. Then all you deal with are the instruments. You have to unpack them and set them out for the surgeon. Once the instruments are sorted, the patient's on the table, the nurse passes the instruments to the surgeon. If she needs anything that's not in reach she calls the circulating [run-around] nurse who fetches it and opens up the pack and has a particular way of passing the instrument without contact.

'Watching it, you think, I'm never going to get to grips with this, but you get used to it.'

The physical side of surgery surprised Corinne, as it did most of the students, with its indelicacy. She hadn't expected to be squeamish, but when she saw the orthopaedic surgeon using hammers to do a knee replacement, she was shocked. 'It's more like a carpentry lesson than anything else.' However, that too was something she found she got used to.

The first few times she acted as a scrub nurse, Corinne concentrated so hard on her tasks that she saw little of the operation. Gradually, though, she was able to take in the broader picture as she had been doing when only observing. She was particularly interested in Caesarean sections and was lucky to be present at several. The atmosphere at Caesareans was quite different from that at most operations, because the patient was almost always conscious and there was no time to plan and take things at a measured pace. 'You get a phone call saying there's a woman in labour and then it's all rush and panic. Some of the ones I saw were emergencies, but in any case it's always very quick. The longest thing is getting the room ready; once they bring the patient in, it takes about five minutes.'

A midwife was always with the patient, but Corinne never saw a patient accompanied by a partner – though once the patient's mother came in too. The midwife's first consideration was now the baby, so a nurse was assigned to the patient, to talk to her, explain what would happen and reassure her that she wouldn't feel any pain.

'They give the woman a local anaesthetic and put up a cage to screen her from what's going on. The abdomen is opened laterally. There are so many layers – the skin and the fatty layer, then the water bursts, then there's the baby. They really tug away at the mother's stomach; they usually grab the baby from the waist and pull it out. It's scrunched up and its eyes are closed. The midwife is waiting there with the blankets to wrap the baby in.'

Corinne usually followed the midwife, so that she could see how she cared for the baby: clearing its nose, checking that it was breathing independently, cleaning it. Sometimes the midwife had to move fast: one patient came in for an emergency Caesarean because she had an infection. When the baby was taken out, it had a bad smell to it and was rushed into the incubator to be screened and tested.

The unsatisfactory side of being in theatres was the lack of continuing contact with the patient; for instance, Corinne never knew what happened to that baby afterwards. But she had enjoyed learning to work at that fast tempo and it was useful to have a different kind of experience now that the prospect of applying for jobs was looming.

The week before Christmas, Corinne started her penultimate placement: five weeks with a community nurse who worked out of a health centre in the north of Wavetree. This would take her through to the end of January, after which she would go for her last placement to A & E at Wavetree District Hospital.

Corinne was unshaken in her desire to be a midwife and, assuming that she registered in March, would go on to apply for the eighteen months' midwifery course at the Wavetree. Under ENB rules, nurses have to have six months' post-registration experience before they start the course, so in the meantime she would be looking for jobs along with everyone else. If necessary, she could make up the experience with agency nursing but she would rather find a proper job. She was not looking forward to the hunt: 'The job list comes out once a month and someone at the health centre said there were only six jobs going this time. There'll be seventy of us qualifying in March. The community nurse I'm with was really surprised because she said she thought a job was guaranteed for you when you finish the course. It used to be like that, but not now. Even for those six vacancies, they'll be taking applications from outside, as well as from us.'

She was concerned, but in a resigned kind of way immediately recognizable to anyone who has looked for a job in Britain in the last five years. 'I won't start applying for jobs until the New Year, perhaps March. Straight after the course ends my mum's going away so I'll be going home to look after my brother for four weeks. Hopefully in May I'll start something.'

She would be looking to stay in London and would be applying for vacancies at Alf's and the Wavetree. She was more enthusiastic about Alf's because, in her experience, the standard of care was better there. 'All the wards I've been on at Alf's have been "top". Everything's very proper, you've always got to do your best. It's been more nerve-racking on the wards at Alf's than at the Wavetree, where they're more laid back. And at the Wavetree, staffing often isn't so good and morale's sometimes low. Some of the wards I was on at the Wavetree in the CFP, when we changed shifts the nurses would say, "Oh, another day here." Whereas at Alf's when you go in at 7.15 all the nurses would be sitting on the bench ready to start the handover, with a smile, and saying, "How are you . . ." '

'Top' and 'nerve-racking'; 'low morale' and 'laid back'; it was interesting to hear Corinne position herself in relation to the two approaches. From choice she would like to be stretched at Alf's; but she could see a way of fitting in to the less ideal conditions at the Wavetree. It reminded me that I had heard her refer to the care on Bartlett as sub-standard and yet say that she wouldn't mind working there if she had more experience. Corinne is an essentially practical person, who takes situations as she finds them. I could imagine her doing well on Bartlett; I could visualize her just as clearly on a highly specialized 'top' ward such as neurology. Corinne herself would not be drawn further: she was keeping an open mind.

Meanwhile, she had already taken a step away from being a student: she had officially moved in with Harry. She still kept her room on the first floor of the nurses' home, but primarily as a store-room. She was twenty-three now and tired of the restrictions of college living. When I asked her if living out suited her better, she smiled at me as if I were mad to ask.

EMILY'S HOLIDAY had been a world away from the London borough of Wavetree. She and Patrick had gone to Tunisia, on an organized adventure which took them across the desert and to the foothills of the mountains. The trip had whetted both their appetites to return and explore the country at their own pace.

Back at Alf's, she went straight into her elective, on Marlowe Ward. Emily had never been there before and her first impression was 'how small it was compared to other wards. The treatment room's like a cubby-hole. And with everyone in their own rooms, it's quite hard to make contact.'

She was on with another student, her next-door neighbour from the hostel, but apart from the initial day together, they were given a rota of opposing shifts. On that first day, however, they met Liz, who showed them round and explained the principal drugs to them. Liz then went off on a course, and between that, some leave which she took and a period of working nights, her shifts did not coincide with Emily's for the rest of the placement.

It didn't take Emily long to realize that her role was going to be circumscribed. It was the familiar problem of being a student in a highly specialized and well-staffed ward: 'The staff nurses differ in their opinions of what we can do. On the whole they are very keen for you to learn; if you show interest you're given a lot of encouragement. There's reading material and the staff know so much that you can tap into their knowledge. It's just that there's not the opportunity to *do* as much as I'd hoped. You might be given just one or two patients to look after in a shift, and they might need only observations and their drugs checking.'

Drugs were a central part of Emily's work, somewhat to her surprise. After Liz's initial introduction to the drugs used, a routine was established whereby on every shift Emily would accompany a nurse administering drugs. 'You're given the drugs charts and you go round with the nurse and check the drugs, and the nurse explains what it's for, the significance of this drug for this person, what the side effects are and so on. On other wards you don't get the chance to do that.'

Because drugs figure so largely in the treatment of AIDS, this was a useful grounding. It enabled Emily to learn not only about the drugs themselves but about the care involved in giving them and in managing their secondary effects.

'This area attracts me in the same way that oncology attracts me. You are not just worrying about the broken hip: there's a lot of emphasis on psychological care. It interests me I suppose because people are dying and you get the chance to use the basic nursing skills to help them. You can help them have baths, with elimination problems – by fitting catheters and dealing with constipation. Doing things for people which at the end of the day make all the difference when you're dying.'

All the same, Emily found her time on Marlowe frustrating. She kept thinking that this was her last placement on a ward: she would be in the community next and finally in A & E, which she did not really think of as a ward. She would have liked to be doing more for the clients.

She was also slightly self-conscious with the male nurses.

'The men on the staff all seem to be homosexual and I sometimes find the atmosphere claustrophobic, a bit exclusive. Many times I felt in conversation that I couldn't say I had a boyfriend. I felt I had to keep it back that I was heterosexual.'

Emily estimated that at least half the staff on the ward were men (in fact four out of fourteen nurses are male). 'I can see why, because 80 per cent of the clientele is homosexual.' She had no difficulty in talking to the clients; it was the fact that she could see no place for herself in the culture of the nursing team that bothered her.

The positive side of being underemployed was that she had plenty of time to talk to people. She grew adept at going into clients' rooms to do observations and giving them openings for conversation, should they want it. Quite often they did.

'People are much more willing to talk about death or dying than on the other wards. I think that's because the prognosis is more certain. Not everybody dies of AIDS but statistically it's likely. It was really amazing sitting with people and hearing them talk about their partner who died last year, and now they're dying. Someone said, "This time last year I didn't expect to be here. I'm trying to make it to January because me and my partner are going on a cruise around the Caribbean using all my life savings."

'I don't find it very easy to talk to people about death, especially if they haven't brought it up first. Sometimes we skirt around the issue; they talk about "the end" and we never say "death" or "dying". We learn in college about opening things up and helping people find ways to discuss it, but it's hard when there's the real person in front of you. I sometimes hold myself back because I'm only there for one shift – sometimes you feel you help people open up and then walk away from it. You take people's coping mechanisms away slightly.'

She also, she admitted, felt callow in comparison with the permanent team on Marlowe and with the clients themselves. Given the enormity of the situation most clients were in and the 'hours and years', as she put it, that they had been contemplating it, it seemed rather preposterous for a student to come along and offer them a bit of help with the eternal verities.

George was admitted in her third week. He was in his late thirties and came from Wales; he had been diagnosed with HIV several years before and had now developed an opportunistic infection. He had originally been the professor's patient at the west London hospital and had not been in Marlowe before; he had received outpatient treatment at a clinic in Wales, as had his partner (also HIV positive), and they were both staggered at the freedom and acceptance of their condition which reigned here.

'When Alan, his partner, came to visit him, he couldn't believe it. He was tiptoeing around. George said, "Let's go to the kitchen and make a cup of coffee." Alan said, "You can't do that!" Apparently there's a very backward attitude even in some of the hospitals in Wales; he said people would throw their hands up in horror if they knew what was the matter with him. Alan keeps saying he's going to get his care here too, when he gets ill.'

George and Alan had been partners for years, but hadn't come out to George's family. George's mother was elderly and widowed and George had been trying to protect her, both from the shock he thought his sexuality would give her and from the knowledge of his condition. So, although some of George's brothers and sisters knew the truth, George and Alan were officially just good friends and had separate homes. None of the family knew he was HIV positive.

Now that George was seriously ill, Alan went to see some of his brothers and sisters, to tell them. They began to visit him, and there was much discussion of who should tell whom and how. Finally all the brothers and sisters knew except one, Dilys: no one had liked to tell her as she was going through the menopause and having a hard time of it. They agreed to bring her up to Alf's to see George, so that he could tell her himself.

Emily was on duty when the visit took place and walked into George's room to do his observations just after he'd broken the news. 'She was sitting on the bed next to him and another brother was there. She was obviously anxious, agitated and upset and she immediately launched into: "I can't believe he didn't tell me! I'm so angry he didn't tell me! I can't understand it – can you?" She was so angry with the shock of it all.

'Poor George was sitting there looking so sheepish, with his sister on one side and his brother on the other. I just didn't know what to say, I didn't feel I could sit down and discuss it, so I said I'd go and get the sister on duty. She came in and got the same reaction, so she persuaded Dilys to go into the office, because George wasn't saying anything, he didn't really want to be in the conversation, and she didn't feel it was fair to talk about him as if he wasn't there.'

Emily did her observations and melted away. She saw Dilys go back into the room and eventually leave, apparently calmer. Later George came out to find the sister and thanked her. 'He said, "Whatever you said, it was brilliant. She really accepted it and it's made a difference." I asked her what on earth she'd said and she explained that she'd talked to Dilys about being George and living in a village, and got her to agree that in his position she wouldn't want people to know. And that had done the trick.'

George was at one end of the spectrum of clients: quite fit, experiencing his first AIDS-related illness, mentally and socially very much in the swim. At the other end was Adrian, who had contracted meningitis and had begun having fits ('fitting' in hospital speak). The fitting had affected his brain in the same way as a stroke might: he had expressive and receptive dysphasia, which meant that he got words jumbled up, both when he tried to speak and when he tried to interpret what other people said to him. He was sometimes confused and disoriented and he did *not* want to be in hospital: he was sectioned in order to get him to stay. This meant that when he tried to leave, the staff could restrain him: 'Not physically, with ties, but stand in the way of the door.'

It was difficult for the staff to nurse Adrian; all the nurses hated the idea of having someone in unwillingly. He needed a lot of drugs, including antibiotics every few hours, which were given intravenously; Adrian would often pull out his cannula half way through the process.

He deteriorated rapidly as well: by the end of Emily's placement he was extremely disoriented. He would wander off and not know where he was; he would urinate in the sink, pour tea on his cereal or try to eat his cigarette. Never having known him before this, Emily struggled to find the right tone in which to speak to him: she was always having to stop him doing things and it was hard not to treat him as a child.

The ethics of whether Adrian should be restrained and treated troubled most of the nurses. Liz (who nursed Adrian during and after Emily's time there) was upset by the need to restrain him but thought that it would have been unfair to let him go home, as he wasn't able to understand that he needed drugs and so would almost certainly stop taking them and die.

Emily thought that given his condition, keeping him alive was not much of a service. 'I think there is a reluctance on the ward to take away treatment before the bitter end. It's not just Adrian – there are some people there who are having treatment which is making them very sick and they're obviously going to die quite soon. There's one gentleman there who's started refusing treatment and refusing to eat and drink. He's the one having to put forward the idea, "I'm dying, enough is enough." I feel the doctors should have been more aware of it before.'

But that raises the question: does a doctor or nurse ever have the right to suggest that a patient give up? Liz believes not: give them the facts, yes; guide that decision, no. In the summer, she had argued that Louis should be encouraged to fight if that was what he wanted. And Emily acknowledged that 'if you don't know how long you've got, I suppose you want to keep treatment going as long as possible.'

An ethical dilemma of a different kind arose over confidentiality, with Fergus. His wife had left him and he now had a girlfriend; because he was afraid of losing her too, he had forbidden anyone to tell her that he had HIV. Under the rules of confidentiality, the staff had to go along with his request. The psychiatrist and the health adviser were both trying to persuade him to use a condom with her, even if he didn't tell her, but he was reluctant because he said that she would suspect something was up. When Emily left, the girlfriend still did not know.

Emily was more cautious about going into AIDS nursing now that she had seen its complexities. 'I was asking, do they employ nurses straight from college, but they said they don't stay very long because it's such a difficult job. The pressures on you become too much. I would love to think that in X number of years it might be something I'd aim towards.'

Emily was very much looking ahead now, and trying to gather up all the things she had learnt. The kind of nursing she enjoyed was on wards with continuous patient contact; she wasn't going to get much of that in her next two placements. She felt that she was going into a hiatus and that the coming weeks would be a matter of holding steady and waiting for things which, when they came, would have a decisive influence on her future: the exam results and the job lists.

JANE HAD REBELLED against the list of elective options: although there were no places left on it, she had written her name against ITU. Whether it was chance or the hand of God, she didn't know, but she had been duly placed there.

ITU stands for Intensive Therapy Unit and is often called Intensive Care. Jane spent the first week of her break in Yorkshire with family, the second in London with friends, and then began on ITU. Her stint on Landor, the general medical ward, seemed to have broken her jinx: once again she enjoyed herself. 'It's very interesting, and though the day is long – you do a twelve-hour shift – you get really good breaks! And you get lots of days off too!'

Jane probably would have had more to say about ITU had I spoken to her at the time, but we couldn't seem to coincide. By the time I asked her about it, she had moved on and was more interested in thinking about her future. She was determined not to join the rush for jobs, she said: 'I think all this hysteria is a shame. I prefer to wait until the end of the course. I think people are getting so worked up, they end up taking things they don't really want, just to have a job. I'd rather wait. Anyway, I still feel like a fraud – I don't really feel that I could do a nurse's job.'

But she wanted to, which was the decisive change. 'Yeah, at last. I was wondering back there, is this all going to turn out to have been a horrible mistake? But I really enjoyed it on Landor and on ITU, and I'm really into nursing now. I think I'll do some agency when the course finishes – I'll see if I can do it on Landor, because I'd really like to go back. I understand the sister there, I can see where she's coming from.'

THE END OF THE YEAR was an unhappy time for Angela. Far from being the reunion she had hoped for, her post-finals trip to America brought to the surface all the strains in her relationship with Mark. Their lives now seemed to be set in two different directions and they agreed to separate.

Angela came back to England with all her plans in disarray, not knowing any longer what she wanted to do.

Her first instinct was to cut herself off from America and her imagined future with Mark; she half decided to look for a long-term job on registration and commit herself to staying in London another year. But at this point she could not think very clearly. It was hard enough coming back to the British winter, which she had always hated, and the room in the hostel, which seemed even smaller than before.

Angela's elective, in theatres, passed uneventfully. She was glad to be able to spend her days concentrating on clinical matters and she opted to spend a good deal of time in the recovery room, in order to overcome her fear of unconscious patients. At the end of her five weeks, she was no longer afraid and she felt confident that she could recognize the signs of a problem in a patient's recovery. Like Corinne, she was pleased to have had the experience but more certain than ever that she would not be working in this field. I had often thought that these two were attracted to midwifery from entirely different angles (Angela's social-political, Corinne's practical and emotional), but in their rejection of surgical work and its lack of human interaction, they were identical.

Angela began her community placement in December. (She was on a slightly different timetable from Corinne's and the two did not work together.) She had expected to hate it, as she'd always found such placements depressing and badly organized in the past. This time, however, she was assigned to a community nurse, given a caseload of patients and allowed to go and see them and give them nursing care unsupervised. The work itself was similar to the kind of thing she had been doing the previous winter: going to flats on the shabby Wavetree estates and changing dressings for elderly people. But the estates were not rough enough for her to feel afraid, and the people, though obviously not well off, were not as poverty stricken as some she had seen.

'I really like being autonomous. I get to decide how I'm going to do the dressings and I get to build up relationships with the clients. You know, it's interesting – I always thought I would be far more clinically oriented, but it's obviously the client contact that I like. That and being able to take responsibility.'

She was not exactly looking forward to Christmas (which she would be spending with friends in Ireland) but she was not dreading it as much as she had been. Like all the other students, she was beginning to feel on tenterhooks about the exam results. They had been supposed to come out a week before Christmas; then it was going to be days before Christmas; then someone heard that it might not be until Christmas Eve. In the end Christmas Eve arrived and the college office closed for the holidays and the students were still waiting. Angela stocked up on cigarettes. 'I've promised myself that when the results come, if I pass, I'll quit.'

JANET HAD RETURNED from her holiday in Crete feeling rested and well. No announcement had been made during her absence about the future of A & E, and none was forthcoming on her return. This caused mild concern among some staff, who still felt in limbo and would have welcomed official postponement of the closure. On the other hand, they realized (with some satisfaction) that the Department of Health must be knee-deep in calculations about the cost and time-scale of reorganizing London's A & E services. Janet half suspected that the matter might be allowed to drift now, with an announcement that closure had been deferred coming later in the year, or perhaps next spring.

With the threat of immediate closure removed from the department, Janet was able to concentrate on its day-to-day business. One pressing task was to implement the controversial 'assessment within five minutes', which the government continued to demand as one of its Patient's Charter reforms. In Janet's eyes, this was primarily a matter of gathering data, not changing care. She was confident that the care was already excellent.

'Patients have always been seen quickly here, I've never doubted that for a moment. The times when they're not, you can explain it. Mostly it's a matter of simply getting people to document things, but that's easier said than done. People aren't used to doing it, they're used to getting on and giving care. I've got to make sure that the time of assessment is filled in on every single patient card, so we can prove what we're doing.'

She set about it by making it a deliberate exercise, involving everyone in the department. 'I've informed people, I've told them that if they don't do this, we're going to be financially penalized. I said, "I know it's a paper standard and doesn't reflect care, but it's what they want so let's give it to them." '

She then spent the next two months bullying everyone over it and going through the cards herself, again and again, finding out times of assessment where they hadn't been filled in and adding them.

The results were fairly dramatic: in September, the number of patients recorded as being seen within five minutes was 19 per cent; by the end of November it was 60 per cent. Together with her staff, Janet set a target of 80 per cent for Christmas and 90 per cent for the end of January. 'It's become a bit of a game now – let's see if we can make the figures better again this month. I think we've done it without decreasing the quality of the care – that was the worry we had, that by emphasizing the five minutes for everyone, you might end up actually giving less good care to some. But I don't think anyone believes that's happened. And people are seen quicker now.'

The patients were often impressed by the speed at which

nurses emerged from the double doors to assess them. Sometimes they had barely had time to sit down after giving their details to the receptionist. They were-less enchanted by the long wait that followed to see the doctor; for that they waited as long as ever, longer, in fact, because so many cubicles were taken up by patients waiting for beds that new patients had to queue up to be funnelled through the remainder.

The beds crisis was now taken for granted by almost everyone in the department. They had ceased to think of it as a crisis; it was simply the way things were. At first sight it appeared paradoxical because hospital figures showed that the number of patients treated by A & E had actually fallen over the last year. However, the number requiring admission had risen steadily, as had the degree of sickness they suffered. As the weather grew colder and wetter, the trend increased.

Janet tried to account for it. 'I'd say that the dependency of our patients has probably trebled. It's partly because we're seeing more elderly people now: the population's ageing and we've got a lot of older people living round here. But I really don't know exactly why it is. Perhaps it's lack of GP support. Or perhaps it's the move towards giving *more* support in the community, so that people keep going in their homes a bit longer and crunch time comes later, when they're that much sicker. But now a lot of people are needing to stay in weeks rather than days. Chest complaints are increasing dramatically: if we've got eight patients in overnight, which we often have, then the chances are that five of them will be chest complaints.'

The staff were now quite accustomed to having anything up to ten patients in overnight; on one particularly bad night in November thirteen patients had slept on trolleys in cubicles.

Janet was also working hard at her access course, which, once completed, would allow her to begin a nursing degree. The work had to be done in her spare time, from books and learning packages which she ordered from the Open University. She enjoyed it very much, which was just as well as it made great demands on time and energy: 'You have to do a series of 3,000 word essays, based on your experience but with theory behind them. So far I've done "Managing Change" – I wrote about the initial assessment! It was *so* therapeutic, it was like Gestalt: you sat it on a chair and said, "I'm not going to be beaten by you, I'm going to write about you now." My next essay will be on managing human resources, which is a huge topic. I like doing academic work and it's very, very interesting, but it requires an enormous amount of time, not only to do the reading, but to work out how to structure the essay. You have to cover the theory and relate it to your experience, and you've got this limit of 3,000 words which is not really very much. But what's really nice is that I've got all the experience there to draw on. I don't think a staff nurse could do this course; it is very much tailored to people at my level, which I enjoy.'

Doing a nursing degree was becoming part of a long-term plan for Janet: she was only thirty-five and didn't envisage staying in her current role, or a similar one, for the rest of her working life. She would probably want to branch out after another ten years, if not sooner.

AT THE WAVETREE District Hospital, Tim (also thirty-five) was finally getting his first taste of A & E. This was his pre-Christmas placement; his elective on the renal unit was due to come up in the New Year.

Wavetree A & E is similar in size and facilties to Alf's, though housed in a more modern building. It serves a different population, however, almost all residential, and with many ethnic groups represented, including large African Caribbean and Turkish communities.

The two A & E departments of Alf's and Wavetree were

no longer so closely linked as they had been a year ago. The impending merger of Alf's with the Thames meant that the Wavetree Hospital was separating out, to stand alone. Moreover, it was working on ambitious expansion plans for A & E, so that it would be ready to take up the slack when the Alf's department eventually closed. Plans for new building work were already in hand and the prevailing feeling was one of optimism.

Tim had been looking forward to working on A & E. It held the same appeal for him as surgery: it was an area in which people got better and in which nursing care could make a swift, visible difference. He was also still interested in the possibility of A & E as a career, or a way into one, but he was well aware that it was a popular choice and that A & E departments did not usually take on nurses with no post-registration experience. 'They prefer nurses with at least six months' experience, because you have to have the confidence to do procedures without looking over your shoulder. That few moments of indecision could make a difference.'

He began the placement with some stirring expectations of bustle, pace and drama. On his first day, therefore, he was surprised by the calmness of all the staff. Another thing that surprised him, though this took slightly longer to sink in, was that the nurses were entrusted with a good deal of initial diagnosing and the doctors listened to them. As time went on, he realized that power relationships in the department were not as he had anticipated: in fact, the doctors were usually quite junior, unless a consultant happened to come down, and the nurses on duty often had more experience not only of A & E work but of medicine in general. The doctors were only too happy to glean some of their knowledge.

On the first day, Tim was still trying to match up the reality with his expectations when he was asked to look after a new arrival. 'This seventeen-year-old lad went to the reception desk and the receptionist came out and said, "Get a chair, quick, this chap is keeling over." Myself and my colleague, Peter, we got him a chair and he was falling off it in agony. We thought he must have an ulcer or something, so we did observations: temperature, blood pressure – nothing out of the ordinary. So we thought he was too ill to stay in reception so we put him to bed in a cubicle. He wasn't made a high priority because there were no physiological symptoms to show that there was anything wrong with him, and if you did have a burst appendix or something like that, your pulse would be racing, your temperature would be sky high. But he was screaming, grasping his stomach. I found it quite scary.

'There were a few RTAs and emergencies came in and they had to be seen first. But Peter and I were both getting quite annoyed with the staff, who were just saying, "Leave him, he's only priority three." And when we said, "But he's in agony," they said, "Look at his obs. Everything's normal." We even did an ECG on him, a heart monitor, and that was perfectly normal.

'After about two hours he said, "I've not been seen yet." I explained that we'd had some RTAs and some people had come in suspended (dead in the ambulance basically) and had to be resuscitated, and I said, "I'm sorry, I know you're in pain, you'll be seen as soon as we can." And he said, "Well, I'm not waiting here any longer," and got up off the bed and walked out!'

Tim and Peter were astounded; the experienced staff were not. They said he had probably had indigestion. Over the next few days Tim saw enough people coming in doubled up with minor complaints to decide that they were probably right. Looking wary and amused at the same time, he suggested there might be a cultural aspect to it: 'This lad was Turkish and I don't want to say naughty things about Turkish people, but I did note that they seem to have a very low pain threshold. It's known that southern European people in general have low pain thresholds, but it seemed there that it was Turkish people especially. They'd be screaming in agony, you'd think their head had fallen off, and they'd have a cut finger.'

The pain might have been real enough to the sufferers, but it bred a certain hardness of heart among the staff. 'Some of them are quite tough towards patients but I can understand that. One lady came in in an ambulance because she had toothache. She was made priority four, the very lowest, and even when the other patients had been seen they still kept her waiting a couple of hours to teach her a lesson. It was explained to her that it wasn't an appropriate way to use the ambulance service – it costs £600 to call an ambulance out.'

The staff's annoyance with time and money wasters was exacerbated by the fact that the Wavetree had its share of real emergencies. Tim admired the way the department clicked calmly into a routine to cope with these. 'There's a red telephone and when that rings it means there's an ambulance on its way. Then you bleep the trolley team which alerts the anaesthetist and general surgeon, who will all be ready when the ambulance arrives. When a suspended arrives, the barrier in the car park is already open for them, so are the doors. They are taken straight into the resus room.'

For all the expertise and equipment, very few suspendeds survive. Most of them have suffered road traffic accidents or heart attacks, and if cardiac pulmonary resuscitation (heart massage) isn't done within ten minutes, there's very little chance of survival. Speed is therefore vital, but usually they reach the hospital too late; in his four weeks there, Tim saw somewhere between fifteen and twenty come in (he lost count), only one of whom lived.

Tim's role on these occasions was that of an onlooker, or someone who helped to prepare the equipment. At the minor injuries end of the scale, he was given more responsibility and carried out inital assessments. 'If someone came in in an ambulance, but the injury wasn't severe – perhaps they'd fallen over in the street – I'd see to it, then someone else would check over what I'd done. I'd do the observations, check the pupils (if they've fallen over you always do that to check that they're dilating properly. If they're not, it could be a sign of brain injury). If they were unconscious you would ask questions of whoever was with them. Check that there was normal strength in the hands and feet – loss of power there can mean brain damage as well. If someone had lost consciousness for any period of time I'd make it a priority two. If someone has a chest pain, you'd do an ECG immediately, that's standard practice. It might be nothing at all but sometimes they've had a heart attack and not realized.'

Once Tim had given a priority to the patient, it would be checked by another member of staff.

Tim's view of A & E made an interesting contrast with Janet's: as a nearly registered student, he brought a fresh and enthusiastic eye to the clinical practice and to the little details of routine which she took for granted. One striking similarity, though, was the speed with which he grew accustomed to overcrowding. Just like its Alf's counterpart, Wavetree A & E had a permanent bed shortage. It dealt with it inventively.

'There's a fairly small waiting room there and almost every day they would close it, move all the chairs out and make it into an extra ward. They'd put beds in there; it could only hold six comfortably, but one time we had ten in there – they were literally next to each other.

'They were real hospital beds but there were no facilities at all. Some of the patients were very sick, too: we had people in there on heart monitors. One, sometimes two members of staff would have to be put on to that ward to look after people, to give them meals and wash them. There was no privacy of course, it all had to be done with roll-about screens.'

Bottomley Ward, as the staff called it, was in use for a

good part of most days. Once it ran for two days continuously while the work of the department went on around it.

While Tim entertained no immediate hopes of a job in A & E, he liked what he had seen of the work and the way the department ran (apart from Bottomley Ward), and he felt he'd packed in more experience in four weeks than might have come his way in months on other wards.

Perhaps it was lucky for him that he'd been sent to Wavetree rather than to Alf's: it meant he was able to leave what had been a good placement on a high note. When I saw him one week before Christmas, he was drinking whisky – a treat on a student's bursary – and making arrangements to go off later with Peter, several colleagues and some cans of beer to see Rory Bremner doing a live show. Along with the other students he had entered the semi-festive limbo of college work, pre-Christmas socializing and waiting for exam results. Yet 400 yards away from his room, Alf's A & E was reeling.

The Secretary of State had just made her announcement about its future. It was to close within ten months, and be replaced by a minor injuries unit.

THE EFFECT of this announcement on Janet and her staff was quite literally stunning. No one had expected it. It was hard to know how to react. 'It was like an earthquake hitting us,' she said afterwards. 'We knew we would close but we thought things would wind down over five or ten years. To hear that the changes would come into effect ten months hence was an incredible shock to us.'

After the initial twenty-four hours of disorientation, during which news crews bombarded the department with requests for interviews and comments, Janet took stock. This was the final decision; there was no point in hoping that facts, figures or representations from interested bodies would alter it. What the department had to do now was take back the initiative and get going on plans for the minor injuries unit. Janet telephoned a friend at a west London hospital where a minor injuries unit had been up and running for a year. She had been intending to go and see the place for months; now she organized an immediate, official visit and took several colleagues along, armed with a list of searching questions about how the place ran, what the problems were, what they would do differently if they had their time again.

It was a very informative meeting and Janet used what she had learnt to produce a document full of proposals for her consultant. He in turn would be using that to draw up an official proposal to go to the district health authorities. 'We're moving very, very fast, because we want to be able to say, "This is what we want to set up," rather than have things dictated to us.'

What they wanted to set up was a minor injuries unit entirely run by nurses, one H grade or equivalent (Janet herself) and the rest sisters. Janet wanted the sisters to rotate between the new unit and A & E at the Thames, spending at least three-quarters of their time at the Thames. This was partly to ensure that the unit staff kept abreast of all the developments in A & E and partly to safeguard the nurses' careers. 'I'm worried that otherwise they could lose out when it comes to future employment. It might be easy for them to get stuck in a minor injuries backwater and to be seen to be out of touch.'

Janet hoped that all the staff at Alf's A & E could be absorbed into new posts at the minor injuries unit and the Thames. For herself, there was no choice: she would put herself forward to head the new unit. 'Other options just aren't there for senior A & E nurses any more – they are losing so many A & Es across London. People are hanging on to their jobs for grim death. To set up the minor injuries unit, I'll train as "nurse practitioner", an intensive course.

There's additional work I can do after that too.

'In the unit, as patients present, I'll assess them, examine them; I'll send them for X-rays if they need it; I'll read the X-rays and prescribe treatment for them. I'll prescribe medication within restrictions: simple analgesia, antibiotics, that sort of thing. We can do all sorts of wound closure, any sort of plastering; things like treating females with urinary tract infections, which are usually quite simple, and tonsilitis; we can do incision and drainage of simple abscesses.

'You're a mini-doctor. It's interesting and challenging. You've got to be very strong because you're all on your own. This gives me the chance to stay very clinical and I know I'm a good clinician and I enjoy that. But I also enjoy the management side and I enjoy teamwork.'

It was a strange Christmas for Janet. She was preoccupied by the task facing her at Alf's and found it harder than ever to get family and friends to understand just how uncertain the future was, not just for herself but for the whole hospital.

Yet back at the hospital itself in the New Year, she realized that outside A & E the implications of the closure hadn't yet sunk in. 'We've grasped very fully what it will mean but the wards haven't begun to think it through. Nearly 80 per cent of their admissions come through us. Once you lose an A & E department, the hospital will die around it. There are no two ways about that – it's happening all over London.'

T HE EXAM RESULTS came out on 29 December. The students had not been able to relax over Christmas, but they were all back at the hospital when the word went round. They made their way to the college office as soon as they could – those on early shifts had an uncomfortable wait. Throughout the day students were turning up to be given the sealed envelope; some opened it on the spot, while others slunk away to find some privacy.

The news was good; gradually it began to emerge that the adult branch students had done much better than in the summer: out of sixty sitting the finals, fifty-eight had passed. The fifty-eight included Angela, Tim, Corinne, Jane and Emily.

Nicola had passed the finals of the psychiatric branch. And Rachel, turning up early and anxious, found that she had passed too.

The adult branch students felt enormous relief. The marking system had seemed capricious after the summer, and they all, even the most confident, had a little stirring of doubt. They celebrated in traditional style, in the pubs.

Nicola hadn't really expected to fail – her record of academic achievement was good – but she felt a frisson that she would now definitely be going to the Grange. It meant that she could go ahead and move in with David, in south-east London. It would be a long commute to the Grange, but there were connubial advantages to set against that.

In Rachel's flat, however, spirits were rather low. The three who had sat the finals had passed and Diane (the student who had been made to leave the course) had persuaded the college to let her take the summer exam for a third time, so she now had a chance of being able to qualify after all. But no one felt much like celebrating.

'It's partly anti-climax,' said Rachel. 'For so long there's always been an obstacle in the way, this exam to do, this project, then another exam. Now suddenly that's all over, but we're still here and we're going to be here until March.'

They were also exhausted: new placements had started the previous week, and Rachel was on the Special Care Baby Unit (pronounced 'skiboo'), which demanded high levels of concentration and endless observations.

For a while, Rachel wondered if the foregoing months had been an illusion and actually she didn't want to be a sick children's nurse at all. But she was reassured when she spoke to some newly registered nurses, who had qualified just six months earlier on the old course. 'They recognized what we're feeling and said that they'd had it too, but earlier on in their course. They all felt at rock bottom two years in, and we worked out that it's got something to do with the way you feel after a certain amount of rostered service. You just get really tired and overloaded and feel you can't take any more. But they came out of it, so I expect we will too.'

She suspected that they would all feel much better if they had jobs sorted out. She had no truck with ideas of waiting quietly for the right job to arrive: she intended to apply in January, as soon as the vacancies became known. 'I think I'll probably apply for absolutely everything. I'd still love to work on Walsh, but maybe not straight away. Perhaps it would be better to go somewhere that's not so heavy for a while, get a bit of experience on a ward where the children aren't all so sick.'

Rachel was ending the year as she had begun it, in a mixture of optimism and self-doubt. The proportions had changed, however: she was much more confident than before and absolutely sure that she had been right to specialize in children's nursing. She had also stopped assuming that she wasn't good at academic work, her marks having consistently proved otherwise. But she remained very uncertain about what the future held; she had seen too many of her friends riding the jobs' circuit to feel sanguine. And the announcement of A & E's closure, while it failed to shake her, was a sign that things were getting no better.

She had a brisk sort of Christmas – just Christmas Day itself at home with her family – then back to work, head down, till she could do something about a job.

IN SHROPSHIRE, Kate was preparing for a change. She was currently working two or three days a week at the district

Hospital, as a member of the paediatric team. This was a case of something good developing from misfortune: originally Kate had been working there as one of a 'bank' of temporary nurses who could be sent to any ward, but in November the hospital had run out of funds for 'bank' nurses. Kate had expected to be out of work but paediatrics had separate funding; when they discovered she was free they promptly hired her.

The children coming in to the ward had the usual range of complaints: asthma, tonsils to be taken out, broken arms and legs, diabetic attacks. Kate liked the fact that the illnesses weren't severe, but the permanent nurses were sometimes frustrated by the fact that very sick children, or those with unusual illnesses, would be transferred to larger hospitals. 'The nurses here are all trained to a very high standard – most of them have trained with specialists – and they know that they could nurse these children, but the doctors aren't specialists so they want to refer the children on.'

Kate didn't chafe against this, as she'd had the chance to do high-dependency nursing in Alf's, but she did find it odd not to know what had become of the children who left. There was one baby who came in with viral meningitis, which can be dangerous and highly infectious. He was put in a cubicle on his own, in an incubator, and Kate 'specialled' him, i.e. was with him constantly, watching his breathing and his colour, checking his pulse, monitoring the equipment. It was stressful work, as she had to keep alert in case he stopped breathing and needed resuscitation; she did it for two days running and found that though she kept going well during the shift, when she got home she felt wiped out. On the third day, the baby was transferred to another hospital; Kate knew that she would hear no more about him and had a moment's nostalgia for the long-running relationships that developed on Howard.

In November, she applied and was interviewed for the midwifery course at the large general hospital twenty miles away from her home. In mid-December, she was offered a place. The course would begin in the second week of January and last eighteen months. Two days later, she was offered a permanent job on the children's ward. The job would be at a higher grade and would bring in more money. It was also a two-year contract which is about as secure as nursing jobs get these days. She was tempted. 'But I really do want to do midwifery and I don't know if I'll get a place on the course later.' Kate turned the job down.

She and Paul had Christmas at home in their new house. Both sets of parents came to them for Christmas morning drinks, then they had the rest of the day alone. Afterwards, Kate went back to her last fortnight of part-time nursing. She was able to get New Year's Eve off, and she and Paul, together with Paul's cousins, went to a ball in a barn. The night was frosty and the countryside through which they drove was very different from London. Kate was optimistic about her new direction.

IN NOVEMBER AND December, while Emily was doing her elective on Marlowe, Liz was doing a course on treatment in HIV and AIDS, run by the ENB in conjunction with a London university. Liz was given ten study days, during which she attended lectures – 'a mix of good and bad' – and study groups, and there were the inevitable projects to do in her own time.

Part of the course was on the ethical questions that arise in HIV treatment, and it focused Liz's mind on something that had been bothering her for a while: the ethics of testing.

'I know that tests have a role in planning for national health and in knowing what to expect to be treating in the future, but on a personal level I think there are real questions to be asked. I wouldn't want one myself: I can't see what use it would be. If it was positive, you'd be constantly worrying.

And it's not as if the test tells you how much time you've got: AIDS can mean dying in five years or in a few months, if something goes badly wrong.

'People who come for tests don't necessarily think they're going to test positive. I'd say that most people do it for reassurance, or because they're not behaving in a "recommended way" and there's a little doubt. But that doesn't mean they've thought through what it would mean to be positive. And though doctors have a duty to counsel people before they give them the test, I think sometimes they don't take as much care as they should.'

She had an argument ('well, – a "discussion" ') with the other people on the course about it. They were broadly in support of tests but Liz argued that she had seen people coming into Marlowe whose close relationships had been shipwrecked by receiving the official definition of 'HIV positive'. It didn't happen so much amongst the white, gay men who made up most of their patients, as they had a certain sense of fighting a common enemy, but she was disturbed by what she was seeing with some of the African Caribbean patients.

'We had one guy in just before I came on the course: a terrible scenario. He was quite elderly and discovered he had HIV when he was being diagnosed for some symptoms and was tested without consent (not here). The medical people gave him the result and counselled him at the same time, but he didn't believe it. He was completely unprepared, he thought they'd got the wrong result.

'Then they tested the wife and she tested positive too. I don't think she ever spoke to him again. She said she wouldn't have him back home; the children were devastated by the shock of it all.

'He came in to be treated for infections and was put on a combination of drugs. Initially our biggest headache was trying to work out where he could go afterwards. I don't really know what he felt about his wife's rejecting him, he didn't show much emotion. He was so shocked and disbelieving, it took him a long time to be able to talk about his condition at all. Eventually he came round to realizing it was the right diagnosis and I think he thought it probably had been a good thing to get the test result, but it should never have been done the way it was.'

The staff found somewhere for him to go but the day he was due to leave he developed a very bad reaction to the drugs and the infections: his skin dried and cracked as if he'd been burnt. He was in great pain and it was impossible to keep him comfortable, although he was given painkillers and his skin was kept covered. He died within a few days, partly because his skin could no longer maintain his body's heat and moisture.

It had been a terrible death physically; to add to that, the man had been rejected by his wife and his relationship with his children had been thrown into turmoil. The Marlowe staff had been trying to make enquiries about the circumstances of the test, but were not getting very far. 'You never do. As a nurse you have a duty not to allow these things to happen within your sphere of influence but there's not much you can do once they've happened elsewhere.'

Testing for HIV without consent is illegal. Technically, it can amount to assault. It is rarely a simple issue, though: there are certain circumstances when a patient can't give consent – perhaps they're too confused – and the doctors can justify their action by pointing to the fact that a positive test would affect the kind of treatment they give. But Liz was worried that too many people were being rushed or coerced into tests.

'He was an extreme case but I think many African people get tested without the full preparation and counselling. People who aren't native to Britain don't always know their rights, perhaps they're a bit more inclined to put themselves in the hands of the medical profesion and take things on trust, and I think sometimes that's taken advantage of. Also it's such a stigma and African people tend to be very reserved and private and retreat into themselves when they're ill. And the counsellors and doctors are allowing that to happen.'

They were allowing it to happen less than before, however; Liz acknowledged that things were improving greatly as people became more aware of the ethical issues in AIDS treatment. But to her mind HIV tests were an overrated tool in the treatment of AIDS, especially as it was perfectly possible for people to be admitted to AIDS wards on the basis of their symptoms, test or no test.

Back on the ward itself, where she was doing a stretch of nights in early December, Liz said goodbye to George, who was well enough to go home to Wales. His mother had now been told about his illness – and therefore about his relationship with Alan – and had been terribly upset, but not horrified as George had expected. In fact, the whole family was being extremely supportive and Alan was finally able to move in with George as his acknowledged partner.

'Alan's giving up work to look after him. He told me he was never very happy there, they abused him a bit I think. They got very upset when he took time off earlier to look after George; I think in a way he's been looking for an excuse to leave and now George going home has given it to him. Before they left they were trying to work out how much money they'd have to live on.'

The ward was quietening down, as it often did before Christmas. People who were well enough to go home for the holiday usually tried to do so, and the staff made the most of the lull, as they knew that in January and February there would be a seasonal influx of people with chest infections.

Adrian was still in, and still sectioned. He couldn't understand why the staff wanted him to stay and kept on trying to leave; to avoid having to block his path physically, over and over again, the staff were giving him sedatives. Liz hated doing it. 'It changes his personality. He becomes withdrawn and childlike and can't really function, and that's sad. You almost prefer him to be outrageous, but he might harm himself.'

Because most of the nurses felt the same way, they tried to alternate periods when he had sedatives and when he didn't. When he wasn't sedated, they needed to have the time to be with him and explain his circumstances repeatedly.

'I think he still understands that's he's HIV, but I can't be sure. Whenever you go step by step through the reasons why he must stay, he says yes and seems OK, but after a short time he'll be back to not understanding again.'

Liz worked for much of the Christmas holiday period, taking Christmas Day itself off to spend with her family and celebrating New Year's Eve with friends. She had New Year's Day off to recover and laze and then went back to work. There was plenty to do: the new ward was nearly finished, way ahead of schedule, and the Marlowe and Microbiology staff were about to start having strategy meetings, to work out how to share management, nursing and beds. They would begin advertising for new staff soon.

Even though A & E was due to close and Liz anticipated that the general side of Alf's would probably wind down fairly quickly afterwards, she was confident that the specialities of AIDS, oncology and cardiology would remain. She would remain with them, for the time being at least. For some time, she had been thinking she might like to branch out into a different kind of nursing one day. But with the NHS in upheaval in London, this was no time to turn her back on a good job. Besides, the next year promised to be an interesting one for Marlowe staff.

*

CHRISTINE SPENT November doing the odd shift here and there on Reynold. They were not full-length shifts and she did not take on more responsibility than befitted a part-time D grade nurse. She resisted the temptation to try and improve the running of the ward and concentrated on her own care. Once in a while she was asked to go and do a few hours on Hamilton, and in any case she went across the landing now and then to say hello to her old colleagues and clients.

She kept up with the news, partly through her visits and partly because several of the nurses phoned her at home to chat. The ward manager still confided her problems, but Christine didn't encourage her and gradually that side of the conversation dwindled.

The patients were quite well, considering that it was winter, though Grace came down with a chest infection. She obviously missed Christine: at the beginning of December she complained to her that the nurses who looked after her now didn't always do things as she liked.

In December, after a month of only sporadic work, Christine was bored. The hospital said that in the New Year, she would be able to count on a regular day every week on either Hamilton or Reynold, but her pension arrangements allowed her to do more, so she contacted Crossroads, a partly DSS-funded charity which provides carers for people at home.

Crossroads is a national charity which operates through local branches. Christine enrolled with four other newcomers and they were given initial training to be carers: they each had some kind of nursing or caring experience and now had some study days and observation trips to build on this. They would be working with elderly people at first; afterwards they might go on to train for working with children with learning difficulties.

Christine began working as carer for two clients: she spent one night a week at the house of each, sitting with them while they slept, helping them to the lavatory when they woke and attending to anything they needed during the night. Her presence offered a night off to the permanent carers, who had to perform these offices alone the rest of the time.

Relief care like this is crucial if community care is to be feasible. Spouses, relatives and friends carry out most of the 'care' given in the community, and do so unpaid. Their own health often suffers under the strain and sometimes breaks down – at which point social services and the NHS have to intervene again. The service provided by carers like Christine is therefore valuable far beyond the hours given and the tasks performed: it offers a rest for the carer, a new face for the sick person, a bit of human contact from outside.

Christine had always tried to avoid nights in the past. She had worried that she wouldn't be able to stay awake and that she would find the disruption of normal hours disorienting. But she surprised herself by enjoying the work.

On Tuesdays she went to Jim and Patricia. A stroke had left Jim unable to get up on his own, though he could walk with a tripod and one person helping him. Patricia, his wife, looked after him during the days and the other six nights a week and a community nurse visited twice a week. Christine sat in his bedroom with him and read and crocheted while he slept; every two or three hours he awoke and usually wanted to go to the lavatory, so she would take him. Sometimes he just wanted to talk. The night can be a low time for sick people, and Christine would chat to him – she sometimes thought he was reassured by the sound of her voice as much as by anything she said.

Molly was a widow, who lived with her daughter. She was more confiding than Jim and Christine learned that she was eighty-four and that originally she'd had two children, but her son had died. Molly had also had a stroke and was paralysed down one side. She was confined to a wheelchair during the day and couldn't get up on her own. She woke less frequently than Jim: usually just two, sometimes three times a night.

Christine found that she wasn't bored and had no difficulty in staying awake for the ten-hour shifts. The arrangement with Crossroads was that she would stay with these clients for three months and then review the situation. Meanwhile, study days were arranged for Christine and the other new carers: they covered things which Christine knew already, like dementia and incontinence in the elderly, but they included some interesting visits to organizations like Age Concern, and one to a home for children with learning difficulties.

It was not the all-involving career she'd had on Hamilton – it was not a career at all. Crossroads employed Christine as a carer, not a nurse, and the pay was very much lower. Commensurately, the work was less interesting, though easier. But there were compensations: she liked being able to limit her working to two nights and one day a week, and to see family and friends. This year, she had plenty of time to prepare for Christmas. Those nurses she had been close to still telephoned her. She still saw her patients on Hamilton, and not only when she was on duty either: during November and December she was invited to a couple of parties and a memorial service on the ward.

Christine also felt an unlooked for sense of release when she was at work: 'In a way, it's a relief for me not to be responsible for the care other people give any more. When I go to my clients' houses, there is only the usual carer, my client and me. And on the ward now, I only give my care, and I don't try to change other people's attitudes towards the elderly.'

As the new year began, however, St Wenceslas started running into difficulties. They had got rid of so many staff that they were sometimes hard pressed to meet the profession's official requirements for staffing levels on the wards.

Early on in January, Christine went into Hamilton twice at short notice, to help get patients washed and into bed. One afternoon the following week, the ward manager told her that they really couldn't manage – they were going to need a trained agency nurse long term, maybe six hours a day, four days a week. And it would be ideal if it could be Christine.

Christine sat very upright in her sitting room, speaking aloud her conflicting responses. Underneath the window, the china horse looked splendid in the winter sunlight.

'I said no because the way I'm looking at it, they are going to use me to run the ward. And I don't want to start that again. But then yesterday I was in Reynold for six hours and they were so busy, the staff nurse there, she was *begging* me. So I said, "No, I will stick to one day a week", but when she needs a trained staff nurse to come on, then I'll do some extra shifts. Being she is short of trained staff. I'll do maybe twice a week. Definitely no more than twice a week...'

Definitely no more than twice a week, of course. Because Christine doesn't want to be involved in running a ward, unacknowledged and unsuppported by management. She's been there before – though last time, she was on higher pay.

Epilogue

TWELVE MONTHS later, as this book was going to press, I caught up with the nurses once again. They were all in work, though many were not where they had expected to be.

Janet Moore was heading up the new Minor Injuries Unit, due to open in a few weeks' time. She had trained as a nurse practitioner and had recruited an entirely new team of nurses, similarly trained, as all the nurses from A & E had found jobs elsewhere. (Many had gone to A & E at the Thames and Janet was still in touch with them.) The Minor Injuries Unit would be operating from the old Alf's A & E site, which had been redeveloped internally. It would be open seven days a week, twelve hours a day. Janet was currently busy training up her new staff and working out protocols for the way the unit would run. She enjoyed it far beyond her expectations: 'It's a very fulfilling, lovely role to have. I'm very much looking forward to the unit opening. There's going to be a whole book in that – but I'll write it.'

With A & E gone, the outlook for Alf's as a whole was dim. Several months previously, the government had announced that it intended to close the hospital within five or six years. The outcry was predictable, but short: no one was terribly surprised. The hospital's general wards were destined to close and quickly; the specialities would survive, but would be moved to the Thames site as part of the 'merger'.

Liz Howlett was still working on Marlowe. The ward's remit had changed as pressure on the department increased. At the start of the year, the new purpose-built immunology and infection control ward had opened, with certain of its beds allocated to AIDS patients. This was just as well, as the cutting of general medical beds in the hospital meant that soon Marlowe had to find room for non-AIDS patients who couldn't be fitted in elsewhere. There was, in particular, a surplus of patients with infectious conditions, so in the autumn yet another infection control ward was hurriedly opened, and run in liaison with Marlowe. Liz's work now involved much shuttling between the different wards. 'It hasn't been bad actually – it's surprising how adaptable people are. It certainly isn't boring.'

Christine Carton was still working as a night-time carer for her two patients. She was also still employed as an agency nurse at St Wenceslas. She had worked on several different wards since starting on Reynold, filling in where staff shortages were most acute. She could have worked many more hours had she chosen, but she kept her resolution: most weeks saw her doing just one shift, though now and again it crept up to two. I had to get most of this information from a colleague at St Wenceslas, for Christine herself was in Dominica. Unfortunately, she was not on holiday: her father had just died and she had gone home to be with her family.

Catherine Ford was still at the Link. She was now an established member of staff and said that work was going very well; she had no immediate plans to move. Her health was still up and down: she had been diagnosed as having fibromyalgia, a condition that causes aches and fatigue, and had been having acupuncture without notable results. She was often very tired, but she felt under less stress than before. Bob had a new job – not in the community but as charge nurse on an acute psychiatric ward. He was currently acting ward manager, which meant a lot of work but was a good promotion for him. He still worked shifts, as opposed to Catherine's nine to five, but life was manageable and Catherine was 'feeling much more philosophical these days'.

Kate Marshall was one year into her midwifery course in

Shropshire and 'loving it'. She was very busy with course work and placements, had no regrets whatsoever about moving out of nursing, but was slightly pessimistic about job prospects. 'Things around here at the moment are like they were in London when I left. All the hospitals have become trusts, so it's definitely saving money time. But I've been through it before and come out the other side, so I don't let it get me down too much.'

Nicola Darke had joined Catherine at the Link. After six months, she had felt that the Eating Disorders Unit at the Grange was too specialized, and that there wasn't enough supervision for a newly registered nurse. She had joned the Link as a staff nurse in October. She was on a one-year contract, replacing a nurse who was away on a course, and who might decide not to return. At the turn of the year she was enjoying the work very much. She and David had decided to get married the following summer.

Immediately after registering, Rachel Barlow had taken a staff nurse post on Howard. She was kept very busy: Alf's was finding it hard to attract nurses to its general wards and Howard had some severe staffing problems. There was a benefit for Rachel – she gained good experience and was given responsibility early. Nine months after joining the ward, she was preparing for an interview to be made up to E grade. 'I've smoked about twenty cigarettes already,' she said (at eleven am). 'I'm so nervous. But I've had a look at the new off duty and judging by all the things they've got me down for, they've decided to give it to me.' Her personal life was good: for much of the year, Rachel had been going out with Jonathan, a young army officer. He had just started a four month tour of duty in Bosnia. 'It was lovely before he went away, but we'll just have to see how it goes,' she said, resolutely irresolute as ever.

After registration, Tim Russell had joined Alf's renal unit on a six-month contract; that contract had now been extended indefinitely. In the summer he had taken a haemo-dialysis course and since then he'd worked in small, satellite haemodialysis units in far-flung parts of the Alf's catchment area. He enjoyed the autonomy and the chance to develop his skills. At the end of the year he moved back to the acute renal ward at Alf's, where his patients included people having transplants. Tim had been hoping to begin a six-month renal specialist course in April; once he'd done that, he would become an E grade, able to apply for senior staff nurse jobs. Unhappily, he too now suffered a family bereavement. He spent the Christmas and New Year period with his family in Scotland and decided that in the circumstances he did not want to commit himself to a long course of study. He planned to enrol for a later course, in September; meanwhile he wanted to be flexible, so that he could go home more often.

Corinne Turner was working on Greville neurology ward. She had joined it after registration, spent some of the summer 'on loan' to a busy surgical ward, and then returned to spend autumn and winter as a regular member of Greville staff. Along with the other nurses, she worked in rotation on all the different parts of the ward, including recovery. It was extremely busy, which suited her. However, she was not tempted to abandon her ideas of midwifery for general adult nursing. She applied to join the Wavetree's eighteen-month midwifery course and was accepted. She would be starting in April and was looking forward to it.

Angela Torrence was in California. She had returned there in the summer and since then she had been working as a nurse in women's health. She enjoyed it, and intended to continue general nursing for a while before applying to train as a midwife. She also enjoyed being back in America – she was with old friends; she was earning decent money and, of course, this year she didn't have to contend with the English weather.

Jane Riddington was working on a surgical cardio-thoracic

ward in a London hospital that specialized in chest problems. She had gone there in September and was on a six-month contract, which she hoped would be extended. She liked the work and was hoping to do a cardio-thoracic course, which would allow her to apply for more senior jobs in the area.

Emily Mallinson was working on a busy surgical ward at Wavetree. It was not a discipline she had expected to enjoy but now that she'd found her feet, it was going very well. The ward was general surgical, but many of the patients had gastro-intestinal cancer and were in for bowel surgery; there was therefore a link with the kind of cancer nursing she was interested in doing long-term. Moreover, the Wavetree was a good place to be at the moment: it was now independent of Alf's and expanding fast to take up the slack when Alf's closed. All the same, Emily wanted to pursue her interest in working with the dying, and she intended to apply for a job in oncology, or perhaps in a hospice, in the spring.

Appendix

NURSES GRADES AND RATES OF PAY AT THE TIME OF PRINTING

Project 2000 students receive a non-means-tested bursary:

In London	£5,075 per year	(students under 26 at start of course)
	£5,615 per year	(students over 26 at start of course)
Outside London	£4,320 per year	(students under 26 at start of course)
	£4,860 per year	(students over 26 at start of course)

Students cannot claim extra allowances for working unsocial hours.
(Additional allowances are payable to students with dependants.)

Qualified nurses receive a basic salary within a certain range, according to their grades:

D grade	(newly registered staff nurse)	£10,980–£12,585 p.a.
E grade	(experienced staff nurse)	£12,585–£14,565 p.a.
F grade	(sister/charge nurse in charge of ward and staff)	£13,955–£17,085 p.a.

G grade (sister/charge nurse in charge of large ward or department) £16,445–£19,030 p.a.

Extra is paid for unsocial hours, e.g.: evenings, weekends and nights.

Supplements are payable to nurses working in London, up to £2,550.p.a.

The G grade is the minimum for community nurses, community midwives, health visitors, community psychiatric nurses and community mental handicap nurses.

Senior Nursing Posts

Senior clinical posts, involving responsibility for clinical management of a group of wards or a department or a specialist clinical practice are paid in the range £18,370–£23,040 p.a.

Nurse educationalists, whose responsibilities might range from classroom teaching through to budgetary and managerial control of a college, receive between £18,420 and £37,760.

Management posts associated with nursing can attract salaries of up to £35,000 at hospital level and up to £45,000 at regional level.

(This information is taken from leaflet HSC10 in the Health Service Careers series, available from the English Nursing Board (ENB), the Department of Health and the Central Office of Information.)

Index

Aballa, Mrs, 121, 241
Accident & Emergency (A & E)
 and drug overdoses, 188, 256–60
 meeting of senior nurses, 157–9
 and the Patients' Charter, 157–9, 313–14
 Rachel Barlow on district hospital placement, 188–9
 St Alphege's, 29, 87, 98–107, 153–66, 253–60, 312–15
  bed shortages, 99–100, 314
  doctors, 92, 101–2
  and GP referrals, 156–7
  and major incidents, 159–62
  as minor injuries unit, 157, 320–2
  patient characteristics, 97–9
  patients needing wards, 99–100
  patients' order of priority, 91–2
  and the press, 96
  and road traffic accidents (RTAs), 97, 98
  seasonal patterns of patients, 98–9
  and social services, 98
  staff shortages, 96–7, 254–5
  threatened closure, 155–6, 253–4, 312–15, 320–2
  and the treatment of trauma, 94
 suspended cases, 317, 318
 Wavetree District Hospital, 315–20

Adam (teenage stoma patient), 127, 128, 130, 131
adolescents
 Rachel's feelings for, 54–5, 127
 stoma patients, 125–9, 130–1
 and tonsilectomy operations, 44–5
Adrian (AIDS patient), 307–9, 329–30
African Caribbeans
 AIDS patients, 141, 327–9
 mental health patients, 72
 nurses, 24, 191
 see also Turner, Corinne
Age Concern, 234, 237, 333
Age Exchange, 234
agency work
 by student nurses, 10, 35
 and Rachel Barlow, 22, 54–5
AIDS
 and drug therapy, 145–6, 150, 304
 and Hickman lines, 147–8, 149
 and HIV, 143–4
 HIV testing, 327–9
 Marlowe Ward, 29–30, 139–53, 245–53, 303–9
 nurses specializing in, 140–1
 relatives/partners of patients, 146, 149, 151–3, 249–51, 252, 306–7, 329
 social class of patients, 143
 see also Marlowe Ward
Alexandra Hall, 20–1

INDEX

Alice (nurse on Hamilton Ward), 265–8
Alice (student nurse in Casualty), 104
amputations, and diabetic patients, 220, 273
Andrew (senior nurse on Marlowe Ward), 246
aneurysms, 174, 177–8, 179
anorexia, 72, 287, 288–91
Avril (Casualty patient), 163, 164, 165

Barlow, Rachel (student nurse), 20–3, 51–8
  A & E placement, 188–9, 258
  and adolescents, 54–5, 127
  agency work, 22, 54–5
  and the CFP, 21, 22
  examinations, 199, 283
  on Howard Ward, 132–9, 189, 201, 233–4
  at Oak Manor school, 55–8
  'obspar' placements, 21–2
  placement with school nurse, 52, 53
  placements with health visitors, 22–3, 52
  primary school placement, 53
  secondary school placement, 54
  and the Special Care Baby Unit, 323–4
  on Walsh Ward, 189, 277–84
Bartlett Ward (orthopaedic ward), 270, 271–2, 302–3
Becky (staff nurse on Casualty), 165–6
behaviour therapy, 182, 290
Bernard (AIDS patient), 146, 150–1
blind children, Oak Manor school for, 55–8
Bottomley Ward, 319–20
bowel diseases, on Howard children's ward, 32–3, 37–40, 41, 43, 124–31
brain disorders, on Greville neurology ward, 174–80
Brian (leukaemia patient), 169–71
Buddhism, and Jane, 24, 25
bulimia, 288–90

Caesarian sections, 300–1
cancer
  adjunct therapy, 225
  deaths, 171–3, 226–7
  Fredericks Ward, 224–8
  leukaemia patients, 54–5, 168, 169–71, 173–4
  Preston Ward, 54–5, 147, 166–74, 225
  radiotherapy, 225, 226, 278
  remission, 169, 170–1
  Walsh Ward, 32, 36–7, 132, 189, 230–1, 277–84
  see also chemotherapy
CAPD (Continuous Ambulatory Peritoneal Dialysis), 218–19, 220, 221
care in the community, 4
  Crossroads, 331–3
  and the elderly, 65, 68
  and mental health nursing, 86–7
  CPNs, 180–7
  see also Link, The
care plans, 50
Caroline (hysterectomy patient), 63
Carton, Christine (enrolled nurse), 30–1, 234–41, 331–4
  as agency nurse, 268–9

INDEX

as Crossroads carer, 331–3
EBN course, 113
on Hamilton Ward, 30–1, 107–23, 189–90, 234–8, 264–8, 333–4
leaves St Wenceslas, 239–41, 264–9
relations with other nurses, 121–3, 264–8
and the RGN conversion course, 31, 121
training and experience, 109–10
Casualty *see* Accident & Emergency
CFP (Common Foundation Programme), 3–4, 5
and Angela, 9–10
and Corinne, 27
and Emily, 11, 12–13
and Nicola, 18, 20
'obspar' placements, 4, 10, 29, 78
and Rachel, 21, 22
and Tim, 15, 16
CFS (chronic fatigue syndrome), 72
charge nurses, grading, 6
chemotherapy, 36, 169, 174, 225, 226
and blood cancers, 167, 169, 170
children's, 230, 278–81, 282, 284
and Hickman lines, 148, 168, 170, 279
mouth assessments, 280–1
and remission, 170–1
child abuse, 135–8, 228–9
children
with learning difficulties, 55, 333
leisure activities, 53
Oak Manor school for blind and visually impaired, 55–8
with special needs, 55
children's (paediatric) nursing, 11, 45–6

bowel diseases, 32–3, 37–40, 41, 43, 124–31, 233
brain tumours, 57
cancer *see* Walsh Ward
care plans, 50
children's illnesses, 40
and drug administration, 46–8
and 'inappropriate' behaviour by children, 229–30
Kate Marshall in Shropshire, 325
tonsilectomies, 32, 41–5, 124
ward schools, 41
see also Howard Ward; Walsh Ward
CMV (cytomegalovirus), 143, 144, 149
cognitive therapy, 182, 290
community *see* care in the community
community nurses, 5, 301, 302, 311–12
CPNs (Community Psychiatric Nurses), 5, 87, 180–8
and drug administration, 185–6
and social control, 185
Crohn's Disease, 37–40, 43, 49, 124–5, 130, 217
Crossroads care scheme, 331–3

Danny (patient at The Link), 206, 215–17
David (AIDS patient), 146–9
day surgery, 88
depression
mental health patients, 30, 72, 78, 82–4, 286
and time management groups, 208–9
Derek (cancer patient), 172–3
diabetes, and kidney failure, 219–20

INDEX

Diole (patient with brain tumour), 248–9
discharge planning, 66, 88, 271
doctors
  and Accident & Emergency, 92, 93–4, 316
  and Marlowe Ward, 248–9
  Tim Russell on, 221, 275–6
Drake, Nicola (student nurse), 17–20
  and the CFP, 18, 20
  examinations, 215
  at the Link, 201, 207, 210–15, 236, 242, 244–5
  on Morris Ward (St Wenceslas), 77–87
  placement with Community Psychiatric Nurse, 87, 180–8
  at The Grange, 20, 85–6, 245, 285–91, 323
dying patients, 141, 167
  AIDS, 305–6, 308–9
  cancer, 171–3, 226–7

eating disorders, 72
Eating Disorders Unit, at The Grange, 286, 287–91
Ecstasy, 256–7
Edie (Hamilton Ward patient), 111, 123, 189, 190, 191, 238, 241
Edward (AIDS patient), 151–3
elderly care
  and African Caribbean nurses, 191
  and Angela, 10–11
  buying extras for patients, 114–15
  Crossroads, 331–3
  day centre for dementia sufferers, 20
  dementia patients, 84–5
  discharge planning, 66, 88
  Leonard Ward, St Alphege's, 64–9
  mental stimulation, 116
  Morris ward, St Wenceslas, 77–86
  nursing homes, 108
  reminiscence therapy, 85, 193–4, 197, 235–7, 268
  Reynold Ward, St Wenceslas, 268–9, 334
  underfunding and understaffing, 65
  validation therapy, 195, 238
  see also Hamilton Ward
elderly care (Hamilton Ward, St Wenceslas), 30–1, 107–23
Elizabeth (patient at The Link), 206, 216, 293–4
Ellis, P. (Casualty patient), 103, 104, 105–7
Emerson ward, 270, 275–6
ENB (English Nursing Board), 6
enrolled nurses, 48
  conversion course for, 31, 48, 121, 153–4, 238, 239, 240
  phasing out of, 239–41, 266
  see also Carton, Christine
ENT (Ear, Nose and Throat) Ward, 270, 274–5
Esther (Casualty patient), 163–4
examinations, 199–200

Fairbrother renal ward, 201, 217–22, 298
Felicity (patient at The Link), 206, 215
Fergus (AIDS patient), 309
Flossie (diabetic patient), 273
Ford, Catherine (staff nurse), 30, 69–77, 291–7
  holiday, 204, 291–2

INDEX

at the Link, 201–10, 213, 215–17,
    242–4, 292–7
Fredericks Ward (oncology ward, St
    Alphege's), 224–8
Fussell general medical ward, 270,
    272–4

George (AIDS patient), 306–7, 329
GPs (general practitioners), 30
    and Casualty departments, 97, 98,
        156–7
    mental health patients, 72, 183,
        186
    and practice nurses, 16
Grace (Hamilton Ward patient),
    111, 123, 189–90, 196–8,
    235, 236, 237, 241
Grange, the (private hospital)
    Alcohol Treatment Unit, 286
    Eating Disorders Unit (EDU),
        286, 287–91
    Nicola Drake's placements, 20,
        85–6, 245, 285–91, 323
Green, Mrs (mental health patient),
    80–2, 187–8
Greville Ward (neurology ward, St
    Alphege's), 166, 174–80

Hamilton Ward (elderly women's
    ward, St Wenceslas), 30–1,
    107–23, 189–98, 234–8
    Christine leaves, 264
    Christine returns to, 331, 333–4
    layout, 110–11
    named nursing policy, 111, 113
    patients' outings, 116–17, 197,
        237
    team working on, 111, 113
health model, 12–13
health visitors, 5

Rachel's placement with, 22–3, 52
Heath Hall (private hospital), 60–3
Heidi (anorexic patient), 289–90
Helen (Casualty sister), 102, 104
Helen (staff nurse at The Link),
    203, 243, 245
Hickman lines, 147–8, 149, 167,
    168, 170, 279
HIV *see* AIDS
holistic care, 12–13, 62, 63
Holly (ward manager of The Link),
    203
hours of work *see* working hours
Howard Ward (children's ward, St
    Alphege's)
    and accident prevention, 135
    bowel diseases, 32–3, 37–40, 41,
        43, 124–31
    Kate Marshall on, 31, 32–3,
        36–51, 124–31, 138, 228–31
    Rachel Barlow on, 132–9, 189,
        201, 233–4
    tonsilectomies, 32, 41–5, 124
Howlett, Liz (sister), 29–30
    and ethical questions in HIV
        treatment, 326–9
    on Marlowe Ward, 29–30, 139–53,
        245–53, 303, 304, 308,
        329–30

Ilana (patient at The Link), 206,
    217, 294–5
ITU (Intensive Therapy Unit), 142,
    310

Jean (doctor), 248–9
Jennifer (Hamilton Ward nurse),
    190–1
Jim (Crossroads patient), 332, 333
Joanne (anorexic patient), 289

INDEX

John (charge nurse of The Link), 203, 207, 210–11, 213–14, 217, 236
John (teenage stoma patient), 130–1
Judy (staff nurse on Greville ward), 175
Julie (child patient), 135–8, 139, 228–9

Kaposi's Sarcoma, 143, 144, 151
Kay (neurology patient), 177–8, 179
kidney failure, patients with, 217–22
Kitty (elderly patient), 65–8

Landor Ward, Wavetree District General Hospital, 223–4
Lena (Hamilton Ward patient), 111, 112, 117–20
Leonard Ward (elderly care ward, St Alphege's), 64–9
leukaemia patients, 54–5, 168, 169–71, 173–4
  children, 278, 282
Liam (neurology patient), 177
Link, The (St Wenceslas), 202–17
  assertiveness groups, 203, 206, 208, 210, 211, 215, 243
  awareness group, 211–12, 243
  Catherine Ford at, 202–10, 213, 215–17, 242–4, 292–7
  drama therapy, 203, 207, 210–11, 243
  men's groups, 210, 293
  Nicola Drake at, 201, 207, 210–15, 236, 242, 244–5
  relaxation groups, 207–8, 210, 216, 242, 243, 292
  stress management, 210, 216, 243
  time management groups, 208–9, 210, 212, 213, 242–3
  women's groups, 208, 210, 211, 243
Louis (AIDS patient), 251–2
Lucy (youth trainee), 191

major incidents (m.i.'s), and St Alphege's A & E, 159–62
Malcolm (charge nurse on Wilcox Ward), 71, 74, 75, 204, 207
male nurses, 16
Mallinson, Emily (student nurse), 11–14, 25
  on Bartlett ward, 270
  and the CFP, 11, 12–13
  ENT, 201
  examinations, 199, 200
  holiday, 303
  on Marlowe Ward, 298, 303–9, 326
  maternity ward placement, 61
  on Preston Ward, 166–74, 225
Mandy (child cancer patient), 282, 284
Margaret (Hamilton Ward patient), 111, 112–13, 120
Mark (staff nurse on Marlowe Ward), 247–8, 249, 252–3
Markham Hospital, 5, 166, 217, 270–1
Marlowe Ward (AIDS)
  Emily Mallinson on, 303–9, 326
  Liz Howlett on, 29–30, 139–53, 245–53, 303, 304, 308, 329–30
  male nurses on, 304
Marshall, Kate (staff nurse), 31, 32–51, 228–32

INDEX 349

on Howard Ward, 31, 32–3,
  36–51, 124–31, 138, 228–31
and midwifery, 35, 36, 263, 325–6
move to Shropshire, 231–2, 260–3
nursing in Shropshire, 262–3,
  324–6
wedding, 260–1
Mary (Hamilton Ward patient), 192,
  193, 198, 237, 241
MAST (Medical Anti-Shock)
  Trousers, 93–4, 95
maternity leave, 254–5
mental health nursing, 11, 30, 77
  behaviour therapy, 182, 290
  and care in the community, 184–5
  and Catherine Ford, 69–77
  cognitive therapy, 182, 290
  CPNs (Community Psychiatric
    Nurses), 5, 87, 180–8
  diagnosis-led approach to, 187
  and medication, 186
  Morris Ward (St Wenceslas),
    77–86
  questioning aspects of care, 86
  sectioning patients, 80, 308
  and social control, 185
  at The Grange, 20, 85–6, 245,
    285–91
  and the 'worried well', 184
  see also Link, the; Wilcox Ward
mental illness, relativist approach
  to, 18–19
Michael (patient at the Link),
  211–12
Michael (teenage stoma patient),
  127–9, 131
midwifery
  and Angela Torrence, 8–9, 59–60
  and Corinne Turner, 25, 26–7,
    59–60, 301–2

and Kate Marshall, 35, 36, 263,
  325–6
midwives
  and Caesarian sections, 300–1
  and student nurses, 59–60, 69
Miller, Miss, 238
Miriam (Community Psychiatric
  Nurse), 180–7
Molly (Crossroads patient), 332–3
Moore, Janet (sister), 29, 90–101,
  153–66, 253–60, 312–15,
  320–2
  access course, 314–15
  and health education, 257–8, 259
  holiday, 260, 312
  job reassessment, 255
  and the minor injuries unit,
    321–2
  and site cover, 95–6, 255
  teaching, 154–5
Morris Ward (elderly mental health
  ward, St Wenceslas), 77–86,
  187–8
MRSA (Methicillin-Resistant
  Staphylococcus Aureus),
  83–4

named nurse policy, 72–3, 268
  on Hamilton Ward, 111, 113
Natalie (psychiatrist), 247
NHS (National Health Service)
  Angela Torrence's attitude to, 274
  Jane Riddington's attitude to,
    274–5
  and the staffing of wards, 61–3
nursing grades, 6, 61, 90
nursing training, 2–6
  degree courses, 34–5, 154

Oak Manor school (for blind and

INDEX

visually impaired children), 55–8
obsessive compulsive disorders, 30, 72, 78, 286
   handwashing rituals, 80–2, 187–8
occupational therapists
   and elderly care, 66
   and reminiscence groups, 85
oncology *see* cancer
operations *see* surgery

paediatric nursing *see* children's nursing
parents, of sick children, 42, 43, 45, 49–50, 128, 129, 131
Parkinson's Disease, 189
Patients' Charter, and A & E departments, 157–8, 159, 313–14
Penny (patient at the Link), 295
Peter (charge nurse on Marlow Ward), 144
physiotherapists, and elderly care, 66
Pitt, Debbie (Casualty sister), 105, 162, 163–5
placements *see* 'observation and participation' (obspar) placements
Poole, Emma (child patient), 38–40, 49–50, 127
practice nurses, 16
pre-nursing courses, 26
Preston (oncology ward, St Alphege's), 54–5, 147, 166–74, 225
Priscilla (college student), 191, 192, 193, 195–6
private medicine, and the NHS, 62–3

Project 2000, 2, 3–6, 35
   and Angela, 8, 9
   child branch and Rachel, 20–3, 51–3
   and Corinne, 26
   and elective placements, 297–8
   mental health branch and Nicola, 17–20
   and Rachel, 21
   RSCN (Registered Sick Children's Nurse) qualification, 36
   specialist branches, 4–5
   and staff on wards, 10, 62
   and Tim, 15
   see also CFP (Common Foundation Programme)
psychiatric nursing *see* mental health nursing

qualified nurses, 6

Rani (Hamilton Ward patient), 111, 112, 114–15
religion
   Emily's Christian beliefs, 13
   Jane and Buddhism, 24, 25
Renee (Hamilton Ward nurse), 191
Reynold ward (elderly care), 268–9, 334
RGN (Registered General Nurses)
   Catherine Ford's training as, 70
   and degree nurses, 34, 35
   student nurses, 27, 64–5, 153, 154
   task-oriented approach, 24
   training course, 3, 4, 5, 21
   and AIDS 142
   see also enrolled nurses
Rhona (mental health patient), 76
Richard (mental health patient), 181–2

INDEX

Rick (cancer patient), 282, 284
Riddington, Jane (student nurse), 23–5
  cardiac ward placement, 166
  on the ENT ward, 270, 274–5
  examinations, 199, 200, 222, 223, 269, 276
  in ITU (Intensive Therapy Unit), 310
  on Landor Ward, Wavetree, 223–4, 310
  theatre placement, 298
RMN (Registered Mental Nurse) qualification, 16
  and Catherine Ford, 70–1
road traffic accidents (RTAs), 97, 98, 317, 318
  brain damage after, 174
Roberta (staff nurse at The Link), 203, 208, 209–10, 212, 243
rostered service, 28–9
Rowena (doctor), 248, 249, 252–3
Royal Marsden cancer hospital, 23
RSCN (Registered Sick Children's Nurse) qualification, 36, 38, 42, 46–7, 133
Rupert French Ward, St Alphege's hospital, 29, 90, 94–5
Russell, Tim (student nurse), 14–17
  A & E placement, 315–20
  and the CFP, 15, 16
  on Emerson ward, 270, 275–6
  examinations, 199, 200, 222–3
  on Fairbrother renal ward, 201, 217–22, 298
  on Leonard Ward, 64–9
  maternity ward placement, 69
  women's ward placement, 166

St Alphege's hospital, 1–2
  campaign to save, 6–7, 87–9, 157
  and Project 2000, 5
  reduction of services plan, 87–8
  see also under individual wards
St Wenceslas Hospital, 5, 12, 77–86
  and Nicola Drake, 19–20
  Reynold ward (elderly care), 268–9, 334
  see also Hamilton Ward; Link, The; Morris Ward
Sally (Hamilton Ward patient), 237
Satira (CMV patient), 149–50
schizophrenia, 19, 30, 75, 184
school nurses, 52, 53, 56, 57
Sevgi (Turkish child patient), 133–5
Simon (child stoma patient), 127, 129–30
Simon (patient at the Link), 213–14, 294
sisters, grading, 6
site cover, 95–6
social workers, and elderly care, 66
Special Care Baby Unit, 323–4
staff nurses
  grading, 6
  pairings with student nurses, 132–3
  responsibilities, 61
  students' relationships with, 47–9
Steven (Casualty patient), 162, 165
stoma operations
  children, 38–40, 124–31, 233
  women's ward, 16
stoma therapists, 126, 128
student nurses, 2–6
suicide attempts, 30, 211–12, 257–60
surgery
  brain operations, 176
  Caesarian sections, 300–1

operating theatres, 134
  scrub nurses, 299–300
  theatre placements, 298–303
Surgery House, 43, 128
Susan (Hamilton Ward patient), 192–6, 198
Susan (sister on Fairbrother ward), 221
Suzanne (Hamilton Ward nurse), 191

Teresa (patient at The Link), 206, 216–17
Tim (AIDS patient), 249–51, 252
Tomlinson Report, 2, 6, 35, 87
tonsilectomies, on Howard ward, 32, 41–5, 124
Torrence, Angela (student nurse), 8–11, 17, 26, 310–12
  acute surgery ward placement, 166, 200
  attitudes to nursing, 11, 200, 273–4
  and the CFP, 9–10
  examinations, 199
  on Fredericks oncology ward, 201, 224–8
  on Fussell general medical ward, 270, 272–4
  at Heath Hall, 60–3
  maternity ward placement, 59–60
  and midwifery, 8–9, 59–60
  placement with community nurse, 311–12
  theatre placement, 298
TPN (Total Parental Nutrition), 49, 127, 130
Tracey (social worker), 211
trauma, treatment of, 94
Trisha (patient at the Link), 295

Turkish patients, 317–18
Turner, Corinne (student nurse), 25–7
  A & E placement, 301
  on Bartlett Ward, 271
  cardiology, 201
  and the CFP, 27
  examinations, 199, 200, 222, 223, 269, 276
  on Greville neurology ward, 166, 174–80
  at Markham Hospital, 270–1
  maternity ward placement, 59, 60
  men's health placement, 60
  and midwifery, 25, 26–7, 59–60, 301–2
  placement with community nurse, 301, 302
  theatre placement, 298–303

Verrey, Hilda (mental health patient), 82–4
Victor (patient at the Link), 212–13, 242–3, 293, 294
Vincent (cancer patient), 171–2

Walsh Ward (children's cancer ward, St Alphege's), 32, 36–7, 132, 230–1
  Rachel Barlow on, 189, 277–84
Wavetree District General Hospital, 5, 82
  Accident & Emergency (A & E), 315–20
  Landor Ward, 223–4
  midwifery placements at, 26–7, 59–60, 69
  theatre placements, 299–302
Wilberforce (mental health patient), 75–6

INDEX

Wilcox Ward (mental health ward, St Alphege's), 30, 182
    Catherine Ford on, 71–7, 201, 204–5
    consultants attached to, 71
    named nurse policy, 72–3
    patient characteristics, 71–2
Williams, Jack, 190, 240, 241
working hours
    days off, 50–1
    nursing shifts, 28